Herbal Face Pack Powder Recipe

Introduction

In today's world, where skincare routines often involve complex products with lengthy ingredient lists, many people are turning to natural remedies for their skincare needs. Herbal face pack powders offer a simple yet effective solution for nourishing and revitalizing the skin using natural ingredients. In this introduction, we'll explore the concept of herbal face pack powders and provide a basic recipe to get you started on your journey to healthier, radiant skin.

Understanding Herbal Face Pack Powders:

Herbal face pack powders, also known as herbal face masks or ubtans, have been used for centuries in traditional beauty practices across cultures. These powders typically consist of a blend of dried herbs, botanicals, and other natural ingredients known for their skincare benefits. When mixed with water or other liquid bases, they form a paste that can be applied to the skin to cleanse, exfoliate, and rejuvenate.

Benefits of Herbal Face Pack Powders:

One of the main advantages of herbal face pack powders is their natural formulation, which minimizes the risk of exposure to harsh chemicals and synthetic additives commonly found in commercial skincare products. Additionally, herbal ingredients often boast a wide range of skincare benefits, including:

1. **Deep Cleansing**: Ingredients like Multani Miti (Fuller's Earth) and neem powder help to draw out impurities, excess oil, and toxins from the skin, leaving it clean and refreshed.

2. **Exfoliation**: Natural exfoliants such as oatmeal powder gently slough away dead skin cells, promoting cell turnover and revealing smoother, brighter skin underneath.

3. **Soothing and Nourishing**: Herbs like sandalwood powder and rose petal powder have calming and hydrating properties, making them ideal for soothing irritated skin and providing deep hydration.

4. **Acne Treatment**: Turmeric powder and neem powder are known for their antibacterial and anti-inflammatory properties, making them effective in treating acne, reducing inflammation, and preventing breakouts.

5. **Brightening and Toning**: Herbal ingredients like turmeric, sandalwood, and rose petal powder help to even out skin tone, fade dark spots and hyperpigmentation, and impart a natural radiance to the skin.

Basic Herbal Face Pack Powder Recipe:

Here's a simple recipe to create your own herbal face pack powder at home:

Ingredients:

- Multani Miti (Fuller's Earth): 4 tablespoons

- Sandalwood Powder: 2 tablespoons

- Turmeric Powder: 1 tablespoon

- Neem Powder: 1 tablespoon

- Rose Petal Powder: 1 tablespoon

- Oatmeal Powder: 1 tablespoon (optional, for exfoliation)

- Almond Powder: 1 tablespoon (optional, for added nourishment)

Instructions:

1. Gather all the dry ingredients in a clean bowl.

2. Mix them thoroughly to ensure even distribution.

3. Transfer the herbal face pack powder to an airtight container for storage.

4. To use, mix a small amount of the powder with water, rose water, yogurt, or honey to form a smooth paste.

5. Apply the paste to clean, damp skin, avoiding the eye area.

6. Leave it on for 15-20 minutes or until it dries completely.

7. Rinse off with lukewarm water, using gentle circular motions to exfoliate if oatmeal powder is included.

8. Follow up with moisturizer or facial oil to lock in hydration.

In conclusion, herbal face pack powders offer a natural and effective way to care for your skin, using ingredients sourced from nature's bounty. By incorporating these simple yet potent formulations into your skincare routine, you can achieve a healthy, glowing complexion while minimizing your exposure to synthetic chemicals and additives.

Orange Peel Powder

Introduction to Orange Peel Powder

Orange peel powder is made by grinding dried orange peels into a fine powder. It is rich in nutrients like vitamin C, antioxidants, and other vitamins and minerals. Orange peel powder is commonly used in skincare and haircare products due to its numerous benefits, including:

1. Exfoliation: The granular texture of orange peel powder makes it an effective natural exfoliant, helping to remove dead skin cells and unclog pores.

2. Brightening: The high vitamin C content in orange peel powder can help brighten the skin and reduce the appearance of dark spots and blemishes.

3. Anti-Acne: Orange peel powder possesses antibacterial properties that can help combat acne-causing bacteria and reduce inflammation, making it beneficial for acne-prone skin.

4. Anti-aging: The antioxidants present in orange peel powder can help fight free radicals that contribute to premature aging, such as fine lines and wrinkles.

5. Oil control: Orange peel powder may help regulate excess oil production on the skin, making it suitable for those with oily or combination skin types.

6. Hair care: When used in hair masks or scrubs, orange peel powder can help cleanse the scalp, remove excess oil and impurities, and add shine to the hair.

To use orange peel powder, you can mix it with other natural ingredients such as water, yogurt, honey, or rose water to create DIY face masks, scrubs, or hair treatments. However, it's essential to do a patch test before using any new skincare or haircare product to ensure that you don't have any allergic reactions. Additionally, if you have sensitive skin, you may want to dilute orange peel powder with other gentle ingredients to avoid irritation.

Orange Peel Powder Suitable for which Skin Type

Orange peel powder can be beneficial for various skin types due to its versatile properties. Here's how it can suit different skin types:

1. **Oily Skin**: Orange peel powder is particularly suitable for oily skin types. Its natural astringent properties help control excess oil production, reduce shine, and prevent clogged pores, which can lead to acne breakouts.

2. **Combination Skin**: Individuals with combination skin, where some areas of the face are oily while others are dry, can also benefit from orange peel powder. It helps balance oil production in the T-zone while providing gentle exfoliation and brightening effects.

3. **Acne-Prone Skin**: The antibacterial and anti-inflammatory properties of orange peel powder make it effective in combating acne-causing bacteria and reducing inflammation associated with breakouts.

4. **Dull or Uneven Skin Tone**: For those with dull or uneven

skin tone, orange peel powder's high vitamin C content can help brighten the skin, fade dark spots, and promote a more radiant complexion.

5. **Normal Skin**: Even individuals with normal skin can incorporate orange peel powder into their skincare routine to enjoy its exfoliating, brightening, and antioxidant benefits.

However, it's essential to perform a patch test before using orange peel powder, especially for those with sensitive skin, to ensure there are no adverse reactions. Additionally, when using any new skincare product, it's crucial to start with a small amount and gradually increase usage to gauge how your skin responds. If you experience any irritation or discomfort, discontinue use immediately.

Benefits of orange peel powder

Orange peel powder offers several benefits for skin and hair care due to its rich nutritional composition and natural properties. Here are some of its key benefits:

1. **Exfoliation**: The granular texture of orange peel powder makes it an excellent natural exfoliant, helping to remove dead skin cells, unclog pores, and reveal smoother, brighter skin.

2. **Brightening**: Orange peel powder is rich in vitamin C, which can help brighten the skin and reduce the appearance of dark spots, hyperpigmentation, and uneven skin tone.

3. **Antioxidant Protection**: It contains antioxidants such as flavonoids and polyphenols, which help protect the skin from damage caused by free radicals, environmental stressors, and UV radiation.

4. **Anti-inflammatory**: The anti-inflammatory properties

of orange peel powder can help soothe irritated skin, reduce redness, and calm inflammation, making it beneficial for sensitive or acne-prone skin.

5. **Oil Control**: For those with oily or combination skin types, orange peel powder can help regulate excess oil production, mattify the skin, and minimize the appearance of pores.

6. **Acne Treatment**: Its antibacterial properties can help combat acne-causing bacteria, prevent breakouts, and promote clearer, healthier-looking skin.

7. **Anti-aging**: The antioxidants in orange peel powder can help prevent premature aging by reducing the damage caused by oxidative stress, such as fine lines, wrinkles, and sagging skin.

8. **Hair Care**: When used in hair masks or treatments, orange peel powder can help cleanse the scalp, remove excess oil and buildup, promote hair growth, and add shine to the hair.

9. **Aromatherapy**: The pleasant citrus scent of orange peel powder can uplift the mood, reduce stress, and promote relaxation when used in skincare products or aromatherapy blends.

Overall, orange peel powder is a versatile natural ingredient that can be incorporated into various skincare and hair care routines to promote healthy, radiant skin and hair.

Side effects of orange peel powder

While orange peel powder offers numerous benefits for skin and hair care, there are potential side effects to consider, especially for individuals with sensitive skin or specific allergies. Here are some possible side effects of using orange peel powder:

1. **Skin Irritation**: The granular texture of orange peel

powder may be too abrasive for some individuals, leading to skin irritation, redness, or sensitivity, especially if used too vigorously or on sensitive areas of the skin.

2. **Allergic Reactions**: Some people may be allergic to citrus fruits, including oranges, which can lead to allergic reactions such as itching, rash, hives, or swelling when using products containing orange peel powder.

3. **Photosensitivity**: Citrus fruits contain compounds known as furocoumarins, which can increase the skin's sensitivity to sunlight and potentially lead to sunburn or skin damage if exposed to UV radiation after application.

4. **Stinging or Burning Sensation**: Orange peel powder may cause a stinging or burning sensation, particularly if the skin is broken or irritated, or if the powder meets sensitive areas such as the eyes or mucous membranes.

5. **Skin Dryness**: Excessive use of orange peel powder or products containing it may result in skin dryness or dehydration, particularly if not followed by adequate moisturization.

6. **Skin Discoloration**: In some cases, prolonged or excessive use of orange peel powder may cause temporary skin discoloration or hyperpigmentation, especially in individuals with darker skin tones.

7. **Interaction with Medications**: Individuals taking certain medications, particularly those metabolized by the liver or affected by citrus compounds, should consult with a healthcare professional before using orange peel powder to avoid potential interactions or adverse effects.

To minimize the risk of side effects, it's essential to perform a patch test before using orange peel powder or products containing it, especially if you have sensitive skin or allergies. Additionally, follow usage instructions carefully, avoid applying orange peel powder on broken or irritated skin, and discontinue use if you experience any adverse reactions. If you have any concerns or pre-existing skin conditions, consult with a dermatologist before incorporating orange peel powder into your skincare routine.

Different types of face pack can be prepared with orange peel powder.

Orange peel powder is a versatile ingredient that can be used to create various types of face packs suitable for different skin types and concerns. Here are a few recipes for DIY face packs using orange peel powder:

1. **Brightening Face Pack**:
   - Ingredients:
     - 1 tablespoon orange peel powder
     - 1 tablespoon yogurt (or milk)
     - 1 teaspoon honey
   - Instructions: Mix all the ingredients to form a smooth paste. Apply the pack to your face and neck and leave it on for 15-20 minutes before rinsing off with lukewarm water. This pack helps brighten the skin, reduce dark spots, and promote a more radiant complexion.

2. **Acne-Fighting Face Pack**:
   - Ingredients:
     - 1 tablespoon orange peel powder
     - 1 tablespoon honey
     - 1 teaspoon turmeric powder (optional, for its antibacterial properties)
   - Instructions: Combine all the ingredients to make a paste. Apply it to the affected

areas or your entire face and leave it on for 15-20 minutes before rinsing off. This pack helps fight acne-causing bacteria, reduce inflammation, and prevent breakouts.

3. **Exfoliating Face Pack**:
    - Ingredients:
        - 1 tablespoon orange peel powder
        - 1 tablespoon oatmeal (ground into a powder)
        - Rose water (as needed for consistency)
    - Instructions: Mix the orange peel powder and oatmeal powder, then add enough rose water to form a paste. Gently massage the paste onto damp skin using circular motions, focusing on areas with rough texture or congestion. Rinse off with water. This pack helps exfoliate dead skin cells, unclog pores, and leave the skin smoother and softer.

4. **Hydrating Face Pack**:
    - Ingredients:
        - 1 tablespoon orange peel powder
        - 1 tablespoon mashed avocado (or banana)
        - 1 teaspoon honey
    - Instructions: Mash the avocado (or banana) and mix it with orange peel powder and honey to form a paste. Apply the pack to clean skin and leave it on for 15-20 minutes before rinsing off with lukewarm water. This pack helps hydrate and nourish the skin, leaving it feeling soft and supple.

5. **Oil-Control Face Pack**:
    - Ingredients:

- 1 tablespoon orange peel powder
- 1 tablespoon Multani Miti (Fuller's earth)
- Rose water (as needed for consistency)
- Instructions: Mix the orange peel powder and Multani Miti, then add enough rose water to make a smooth paste. Apply the pack to your face, focusing on oily areas, and leave it on until it dries. Rinse off with water. This pack helps control excess oil production, tighten pores, and mattify the skin.

Before applying any face pack, it's essential to cleanse your face thoroughly and perform a patch test to ensure you don't have any adverse reactions to the ingredients. Additionally, follow up with a moisturizer suitable for your skin type after rinsing off the face pack.

Rose Petal Powder

Introduction to rose petal powder.

Rose petal powder is derived from dried rose petals that have been finely ground into a powder. It is valued for its numerous skincare and haircare benefits and is often used in natural beauty treatments. Here are some of the benefits and uses of rose petal powder:

1. **Moisturizing**: Rose petal powder is rich in natural oils and sugars, making it an excellent moisturizer for dry skin. It helps hydrate the skin, leaving it soft, smooth, and supple.

2. **Toning**: Rose petal powder has astringent properties that help tone and tighten the skin, reducing the appearance of pores and promoting a more youthful complexion.

3. **Anti-inflammatory**: The anti-inflammatory properties of rose petal powder can help soothe irritated skin, reduce redness, and calm inflamed conditions such as acne, eczema, or rosacea.

4. **Antioxidant**: Rose petals contain antioxidants like

vitamin C and flavonoids, which help protect the skin from damage caused by free radicals and environmental stressors, thus preventing premature aging and promoting healthy, radiant skin.

5. **Cleansing**: Rose petal powder can be used as a natural cleanser to remove dirt, oil, and impurities from the skin, leaving it clean and refreshed.

6. **Exfoliating**: The gentle abrasive texture of rose petal powder makes it an effective natural exfoliant, helping to remove dead skin cells, unclog pores, and promote cell turnover for a brighter complexion.

7. **Haircare**: Rose petal powder can also benefit the hair by moisturizing the scalp, reducing dandruff, and adding shine and softness to the hair strands.

Rose petal powder can be used in various DIY skincare and haircare recipes, including face masks, scrubs, toners, hair masks, and bath soaks. Here are a few simple recipes to try:

- **Rose Petal Face Mask**: Mix rose petal powder with yogurt or honey to form a smooth paste. Apply it to clean skin, leave it on for 15-20 minutes, then rinse off with warm water.

- **Rose Petal Scrub**: Combine rose petal powder with sugar or oatmeal and a carrier oil such as coconut or almond oil. Gently massage the mixture onto damp skin in circular motions, then rinse off with water.

- **Rose Petal Hair Mask**: Mix rose petal powder with yogurt or aloe vera gel to create a hair mask. Apply it to damp hair and scalp, leave it on for 30 minutes, then shampoo and condition as usual.

- **Rose Petal Bath Soak**: Add a few tablespoons of rose petal powder to your bathwater for a luxurious and aromatic soak. The powder will help soften and nourish your skin while you relax.

Before using rose petal powder or any new skincare product, it's essential to perform a patch test to ensure you don't have any allergic reactions or sensitivities. Additionally, choose high-quality, organic rose petal powder for the best results.

Rose petal powder suitable for which skin type

Rose petal powder can be beneficial for various skin types due to its versatile properties. Here's how it can suit different skin types:

1. **Dry Skin**: Rose petal powder is hydrating and moisturizing, making it suitable for individuals with dry skin. It helps replenish moisture, soothe irritation, and leave the skin feeling soft and supple.

2. **Normal Skin**: Even individuals with normal skin can benefit from rose petal powder. It helps maintain the skin's natural balance, tones and tightens pores, and provides antioxidant protection against environmental damage.

3. **Sensitive Skin**: Rose petal powder has anti-inflammatory properties that can help soothe and calm sensitive skin. It's gentle enough to use without causing irritation, making it suitable for those with sensitive or easily irritated skin.

4. **Combination Skin**: Rose petal powder can also benefit individuals with combination skin. It hydrates dry areas, regulates oil production in the T-zone, and helps balance the skin's overall texture and tone.

5. **Mature Skin**: For mature skin, rose petal powder offers antioxidant protection against signs of aging, such as fine lines, wrinkles, and dullness. It helps promote cell turnover, improve elasticity, and maintain a youthful complexion.

6. **Acne-Prone Skin**: Although individuals with acne-prone skin should be cautious, rose petal powder's anti-inflammatory and antibacterial properties can help soothe acne inflammation and redness. However, it's essential to avoid using products containing rose petal powder if they contain other ingredients that could potentially clog pores or exacerbate acne.

Overall, rose petal powder is gentle and versatile, making it suitable for most skin types. However, as with any skincare product, it's essential to perform a patch test before use, especially if you have sensitive skin or specific allergies. If you experience any adverse reactions, discontinue use immediately and consult a dermatologist.

Benefits of rose petal powder

Rose petal powder offers numerous benefits for skin and hair care due to its rich nutrient content and natural properties. Here are some of its key benefits:

1. **Moisturizing**: Rose petal powder is rich in natural oils and sugars, making it an excellent moisturizer for dry and dehydrated skin. It helps hydrate the skin, leaving it soft, smooth, and supple.

2. **Toning**: The astringent properties of rose petal powder help tone and tighten the skin, reducing the appearance of pores and promoting a more youthful complexion.

3. **Anti-inflammatory**: Rose petal powder contains compounds that have anti-inflammatory properties, helping to soothe irritated skin, reduce redness, and calm inflamed conditions such as acne, eczema, or rosacea.

4. **Antioxidant**: Rose petals are rich in antioxidants such as vitamin C and flavonoids, which help protect the skin from damage caused by free radicals and environmental stressors. This can prevent premature aging and promote healthy, radiant skin.

5. **Cleansing**: Rose petal powder can be used as a natural cleanser to remove dirt, oil, and impurities from the skin, leaving it clean and refreshed.

6. **Exfoliating**: The gentle abrasive texture of rose petal powder makes it an effective natural exfoliant, helping to remove dead skin cells, unclog pores, and promote cell turnover for a brighter complexion.

7. **Haircare**: Rose petal powder can also benefit the hair by moisturizing the scalp, reducing dandruff, and adding shine and softness to the hair strands.

8. **Aromatherapy**: The pleasant floral scent of rose petal powder has aromatherapy benefits, promoting relaxation, reducing stress, and uplifting the mood.

Rose petal powder can be incorporated into various DIY skincare and haircare recipes, including face masks, scrubs, toners, hair masks, and bath soaks. It's a versatile and natural ingredient that offers multiple benefits for overall skin and hair health.

Side effects of rose petal powder

While rose petal powder offers numerous benefits for skin and hair care, there are potential side effects to consider, especially for individuals with sensitive skin or specific allergies. Here are some possible side effects of using rose petal powder:

1. **Allergic Reactions**: Some individuals may be allergic to roses or other plants in the Rosaceae family. Allergic reactions can manifest as itching, redness, rash, hives, or swelling upon contact with rose petal powder.

2. **Skin Irritation**: Rose petal powder, if not properly diluted or if used in excessive amounts, may cause skin irritation or sensitivity, particularly in individuals with sensitive skin. This can lead to redness, stinging, burning, or discomfort.

3. **Photosensitivity**: While less common, rose petal powder may increase the skin's sensitivity to sunlight (photosensitivity) in some individuals. This can potentially lead to sunburn or skin damage if exposed to UV radiation after applying rose petal powder.

4. **Clogged Pores**: In rare cases, using products containing rose petal powder with other pore-clogging ingredients may lead to clogged pores or acne breakouts, particularly for individuals with oily or acne-prone skin.

5. **Staining**: Rose petal powder may temporarily stain the skin, especially if used in high concentrations or if left on the skin for an extended period. This is more likely to occur with powdered rose petals rather than commercially prepared rose petal powder.

6. **Interaction with Medications**: Some individuals may be taking medications or using topical treatments that could interact with rose petal powder. It's essential to consult with a healthcare professional if you have concerns about potential interactions.

To minimize the risk of side effects, it's essential to perform a patch test before using rose petal powder or products containing it, especially if you have sensitive skin or allergies. Additionally, follow usage instructions carefully, avoid using excessive amounts, and discontinue use if you experience any adverse reactions. If you have any concerns or pre-existing skin conditions, consult with a dermatologist before incorporating rose petal powder into your skincare routine.

Different types of face pack can be prepared with rose petal powder.

Certainly! Rose petal powder can be used to create various types of face packs suitable for different skin types and concerns. Here are a few DIY face pack recipes using rose petal powder:

1. **Moisturizing Rose Petal Face Pack:**
    - Ingredients:
        - 1 tablespoon rose petal powder.
        - 1 tablespoon mashed avocado
        - 1 teaspoon honey
    - Instructions: Mix all the ingredients to form a smooth paste. Apply the pack to cleansed skin and leave it on for 15-20 minutes. Rinse off with lukewarm water. This pack helps hydrate and nourish the skin, leaving it soft and moisturized.

2. **Toning Rose Petal Face Pack:**
    - Ingredients:
        - 1 tablespoon rose petal powder.
        - 1 tablespoon rose water.
        - 1 teaspoon yogurt
    - Instructions: Combine the ingredients to form a paste. Apply the pack to cleansed skin and leave it on for 15-20 minutes. Rinse off with water. This pack helps tone the skin, tighten pores, and promote a more youthful complexion.

3. **Exfoliating Rose Petal Face Pack:**
    - Ingredients:
        - 1 tablespoon rose petal powder.
        - 1 tablespoon oatmeal powder

- 1 tablespoon yogurt

- Instructions: Mix all the ingredients to make a paste. Gently massage the pack onto damp skin using circular motions. Leave it on for 10-15 minutes, then rinse off with water. This pack helps exfoliate dead skin cells, unclog pores, and reveal smoother skin.

4. **Brightening Rose Petal Face Pack:**
   - Ingredients:
     - 1 tablespoon rose petal powder.
     - 1 tablespoon sandalwood powder
     - Rose water (as needed)
   - Instructions: Mix rose petal powder and sandalwood powder with enough rose water to form a paste. Apply the pack to cleansed skin and leave it on for 15-20 minutes. Rinse off with water. This pack helps brighten the complexion and reduce dark spots.

5. **Soothing Rose Petal Face Pack:**
   - Ingredients:
     - 1 tablespoon rose petal powder
     - 1 tablespoon aloe vera gel
     - 1 teaspoon cucumber juice
   - Instructions: Mix all the ingredients to form a smooth paste. Apply the pack to cleansed skin and leave it on for 15-20 minutes. Rinse off with water. This pack helps soothe irritated skin, reduce redness, and calm inflammation.

These are just a few examples of face packs you can create using rose petal powder. Feel free to customize the recipes based on your skin type and specific concerns. Always perform a patch test before using any new skincare product and discontinue use if you

experience any irritation or allergic reactions.

Multani Miti Powder

Introduction to Multani Miti powder

Multani Miti, also known as Fuller's Earth, is a type of clay that has been used for centuries in skincare and haircare routines due to its numerous benefits. It is derived from sedimentary rocks and is rich in minerals like magnesium, silica, quartz, and calcium carbonate. Multani Miti powder is widely used in various DIY beauty treatments and commercial skincare products. Here are some of its benefits and uses:

1. **Deep Cleansing**: Multani Miti has excellent absorbent properties, making it effective at removing excess oil, dirt, and impurities from the skin. It helps unclog pores and prevents acne and blackheads.

2. **Exfoliation**: Its fine texture makes Multani Miti an excellent natural exfoliant. It gently removes dead skin cells, revealing a smoother and brighter complexion.

3. **Oil Control**: Multani Miti helps regulate sebum production, making it suitable for oily and combination skin types. It mattifies the skin and reduces shine without stripping away natural oils.

4. **Toning**: Multani Miti tightens and firms the skin, giving it a toned appearance. It helps reduce the size of pores and improves skin texture.

5. **Anti-inflammatory**: Multani Miti has soothing properties that help calm irritated skin and reduce redness and inflammation. It is beneficial for treating acne, sunburns, and other skin irritations.

6. **Lightens Blemishes**: Regular use of Multani Miti can help fade acne scars, dark spots, and blemishes, giving the skin a more even tone.

7. **Hair Care**: Multani Miti can be used as a hair mask to cleanse the scalp, remove excess oil and product buildup, and promote healthy hair growth. It also adds volume and shine to the hair.

8. **Cooling Effect**: Multani Miti has a cooling sensation when applied to the skin, making it particularly refreshing during hot weather or after sun exposure.

To use Multani Miti powder:

- For a face mask, mix Multani Miti powder with water, rose water, yogurt, or honey to form a paste. Apply it to cleansed skin, leave it on for 10-15 minutes, then rinse off with water.

- For a hair mask, mix Multani Miti powder with water or aloe vera gel to create a paste. Apply it to the scalp and hair, leave it on for 20-30 minutes, then wash it off with shampoo.

It's essential to perform a patch test before using Multani Miti powder, especially if you have sensitive skin, to ensure you don't experience any adverse reactions. Additionally, avoid using it too frequently, as it can be drying for some skin types. Overall, Multani Miti is a versatile and beneficial ingredient for skincare and haircare routines.

Multani Miti powder suitable for which skin type

Multani Miti powder, also known as Fuller's Earth, is suitable for various skin types due to its versatile properties. Here's how it can benefit different skin types:

1. **Oily Skin**: Multani Miti is particularly beneficial for oily skin. Its absorbent properties help to draw out excess oil, unclog pores, and reduce shine, leaving the skin feeling refreshed and mattified.

2. **Combination Skin**: Individuals with combination skin, where some areas of the face are oily while others are dry, can also benefit from Multani Miti. It helps balance oil production in the T-zone while providing deep cleansing without overly drying out the skin.

3. **Acne-Prone Skin**: Multani Miti is effective in treating acne-prone skin due to its ability to absorb excess oil, remove impurities, and unclog pores. It also has anti-inflammatory properties that help reduce redness and inflammation associated with acne breakouts.

4. **Normal Skin**: Even individuals with normal skin can incorporate Multani Miti into their skincare routine. It helps maintain the skin's natural balance, removes dead skin cells, and promotes a smoother complexion.

5. **Sensitive Skin**: While Multani Miti can be suitable for sensitive skin, it's essential to use it with caution and in moderation. Some individuals with sensitive skin may find it too drying or irritating, so it's best to perform a patch test before using it on larger areas of the skin.

Overall, Multani Miti is a versatile skincare ingredient that can benefit various skin types. However, it's essential to customize its usage based on individual skin concerns and sensitivities. If you experience any adverse reactions, such as excessive dryness or irritation, discontinue use and consult a dermatologist.

Additionally, always follow up with a moisturizer after using Multani Miti to prevent over-drying of the skin.

Benefits of Multani Miti powder

Multani Miti powder, also known as Fuller's Earth, offers numerous benefits for skin and hair care due to its rich mineral composition and absorbent properties. Here are some of its key benefits:

1. **Deep Cleansing**: Multani Miti acts as a natural cleanser, removing excess oil, dirt, and impurities from the skin. It helps unclog pores and prevents acne breakouts and blackheads.

2. **Exfoliation**: Its fine texture makes Multani Miti an excellent natural exfoliant. It gently removes dead skin cells, revealing a smoother and brighter complexion.

3. **Oil Control**: Multani Miti helps regulate sebum production, making it beneficial for oily and combination skin types. It helps mattify the skin and reduce shine without stripping away natural oils.

4. **Toning**: Multani Miti tightens and firms the skin, giving it a toned appearance. It helps reduce the size of pores and improves skin texture.

5. **Soothing**: Multani Miti has cooling and soothing properties that help calm irritated skin, reduce redness, and alleviate inflammation. It is beneficial for treating acne, sunburns, and other skin irritations.

6. **Lightening Blemishes**: Regular use of Multani Miti can help fade acne scars, dark spots, and blemishes, giving the skin a more even tone.

7. **Hair Care**: Multani Miti can be used as a hair mask to cleanse the scalp, remove excess oil and product buildup, and promote healthy hair growth. It also adds volume

and shine to the hair.

8. **Improves Blood Circulation**: Applying Multani Miti to the skin can help stimulate blood circulation, which contributes to healthier-looking skin.

9. **Reduces Puffiness**: Multani Miti has a tightening effect on the skin, which can help reduce puffiness and swelling, especially around the eyes.

10. **Relieves Sunburn**: Its cooling properties make Multani Miti beneficial for soothing sunburned skin. It helps reduce inflammation and discomfort caused by prolonged sun exposure.

These are just some of the many benefits of Multani Miti powder. It is a versatile and natural skincare ingredient that can be incorporated into various DIY beauty treatments and commercial skincare products to promote healthy and radiant skin.

Side effects of Multani Miti powder

While Multani Miti powder offers numerous benefits for skin and hair care, there are potential side effects to consider, particularly for individuals with sensitive skin or specific conditions. Here are some possible side effects of using Multani Miti powder:

1. **Dryness**: Multani Miti is highly absorbent and can draw out excess oil from the skin. While this can be beneficial for oily skin types, it may lead to excessive dryness in individuals with already dry or sensitive skin, especially if used too frequently or for prolonged periods.

2. **Skin Irritation**: Some individuals may experience skin irritation or sensitivity when using Multani Miti powder, particularly if they have sensitive skin or conditions like eczema or psoriasis. This may manifest as redness, itching, or a burning sensation upon application.

3. **Over-drying**: Excessive use of Multani Miti powder can strip the skin of its natural oils, leading to over-drying and potential irritation. It's essential to balance its use with hydrating ingredients and moisturizers, especially for individuals with dry or sensitive skin.

4. **Allergic Reactions**: While rare, some individuals may be allergic to certain minerals or components found in Multani Miti powder. Allergic reactions can range from mild itching and redness to more severe symptoms such as hives or swelling. It's essential to perform a patch test before using Multani Miti powder, especially if you have sensitive skin or allergies.

5. **Sensitivity to Sunlight**: Multani Miti can make the skin more sensitive to sunlight, leading to a higher risk of sunburn. It's important to apply sunscreen and limit sun exposure after using Multani Miti-based products, especially during peak hours.

6. **Pore Clogging**: While Multani Miti is known for its pore-cleansing properties, using it in combination with pore-clogging ingredients or leaving it on the skin for too long may lead to pore clogging and acne breakouts, especially for individuals with acne-prone skin.

7. **Skin Discoloration**: Prolonged or excessive use of Multani Miti powder may cause temporary skin discoloration or hyperpigmentation, particularly in individuals with darker skin tones. It's essential to use it in moderation and discontinue use if you notice any changes in skin coloration.

To minimize the risk of side effects, it's essential to use Multani Miti powder in moderation, perform a patch test before using it on larger areas of the skin, and follow up with a moisturizer to prevent over-drying. If you experience any adverse reactions, discontinue use immediately and consult a dermatologist.

Different types of face pack can be prepared with Multani Miti powder.

Certainly! Multani Miti powder, also known as Fuller's Earth, can be used to create various types of face packs suitable for different skin types and concerns. Here are a few DIY face pack recipes using Multani Miti powder:

1. **Deep Cleansing Face Pack**:
   - Ingredients:
     - 1 tablespoon Multani Miti powder
     - 1 tablespoon rose water.
     - 1 teaspoon honey
   - Instructions: Mix all the ingredients to form a smooth paste. Apply the pack to cleansed skin and leave it on for 10-15 minutes. Rinse off with lukewarm water. This pack deeply cleanses the pores, removes impurities, and leaves the skin feeling refreshed.

2. **Oil-Control Face Pack**:
   - Ingredients:
     - 1 tablespoon Multani Miti powder
     - 1 tablespoon yogurt
     - 1 teaspoon lemon juice
   - Instructions: Mix the ingredients to form a paste. Apply it to the face, focusing on oily areas, and leave it on for 15-20 minutes. Rinse off with water. This pack helps control excess oil, reduce shine, and prevent acne breakouts.

3. **Brightening Face Pack**:
   - Ingredients:
     - 1 tablespoon Multani Miti powder
     - 1 tablespoon tomato juice

- 1 teaspoon turmeric powder

- Instructions: Combine all the ingredients to make a paste. Apply the pack to the face and neck, leave it on for 15-20 minutes, then rinse off with water. This pack helps brighten the complexion, even out skin tone, and reduce the appearance of dark spots.

4. **Soothing Face Pack**:
    - Ingredients:
        - 1 tablespoon Multani Miti powder
        - 1 tablespoon cucumber juice
        - 1 teaspoon aloe vera gel
    - Instructions: Mix the ingredients to form a smooth paste. Apply it to the face and leave it on for 10-15 minutes. Rinse off with water. This pack helps soothe irritated skin, reduce redness, and calm inflammation.

5. **Exfoliating Face Pack**:
    - Ingredients:
        - 1 tablespoon Multani Miti powder
        - 1 tablespoon oatmeal powder
        - 1 tablespoon milk
    - Instructions: Mix all the ingredients to form a paste. Gently massage it onto damp skin in circular motions, then leave it on for 10-15 minutes. Rinse off with water. This pack helps exfoliate dead skin cells, unclog pores, and promote a smoother complexion.

These are just a few examples of face packs you can create using Multani Miti powder. Feel free to customize the recipes based on your skin type and specific concerns. Always perform a patch test before using any new skincare product and discontinue use if you

experience any irritation or allergic reactions.

Neem Leaf Powder

Introduction to neem leaf powder

Neem leaf powder is derived from the leaves of the neem tree (Azadirachta indica), a plant native to the Indian subcontinent. Neem has been used in traditional Ayurvedic medicine for centuries due to its numerous health and skincare benefits. Neem leaf powder is rich in various bioactive compounds, including antioxidants, anti-inflammatory agents, and antimicrobial properties. Here are some of the benefits and uses of neem leaf powder:

1. **Acne Treatment**: Neem leaf powder has strong antibacterial properties that help kill acne-causing bacteria on the skin's surface. It also reduces inflammation and redness associated with acne breakouts.

2. **Oil Control**: Neem leaf powder helps regulate sebum production, making it beneficial for oily and acne-prone skin. It helps mattify the skin, reduce shine, and prevent clogged pores.

3. **Anti-inflammatory**: Neem leaf powder contains compounds like nimbidin and nimbin, which have

potent anti-inflammatory properties. It helps soothe irritated skin, reduce redness, and alleviate conditions like eczema and psoriasis.

4. **Antioxidant Protection**: The antioxidants present in neem leaf powder help protect the skin from damage caused by free radicals, environmental pollutants, and UV radiation. This helps prevent premature aging and promotes a youthful complexion.

5. **Skin Healing**: Neem leaf powder promotes wound healing and tissue regeneration, making it beneficial for treating minor cuts, burns, and insect bites. It also helps reduce scarring and promotes smoother skin texture.

6. **Anti-dandruff Treatment**: Neem leaf powder has antifungal properties that help combat dandruff-causing fungi on the scalp. It also soothes itching and inflammation, promoting a healthier scalp and hair.

7. **Skin Brightening**: Regular use of neem leaf powder can help lighten dark spots, hyperpigmentation, and blemishes, giving the skin a more even tone and brighter appearance.

8. **Purifying**: Neem leaf powder acts as a natural detoxifier, helping to purify and cleanse the skin by removing impurities, toxins, and excess oil.

To use neem leaf powder:

- For a face mask, mix neem leaf powder with water, rose water, or yogurt to form a paste. Apply it to cleansed skin, leave it on for 10-15 minutes, then rinse off with water.

- For a hair mask, mix neem leaf powder with water or aloe vera gel to create a paste. Apply it to the scalp and hair, leave it on for 20-30 minutes, then wash it off with shampoo.

It's essential to perform a patch test before using neem leaf powder, especially if you have sensitive skin, to ensure you don't experience any adverse reactions. Additionally, avoid using it too frequently, as it can be drying for some skin types. Overall, neem leaf powder is a versatile and beneficial skincare ingredient with numerous uses and benefits for the skin and hair.

Neem leaf powder suitable for which skin type

Neem leaf powder can be beneficial for various skin types due to its versatile properties. Here's how it can suit different skin types:

1. **Oily and Acne-Prone Skin**: Neem leaf powder is particularly suitable for oily and acne-prone skin types. Its antibacterial and anti-inflammatory properties help combat acne-causing bacteria, reduce inflammation, and regulate sebum production. Neem leaf powder can help unclog pores, prevent acne breakouts, and control excess oiliness.

2. **Combination Skin**: Individuals with combination skin, where some areas of the face are oily while others are dry, can also benefit from neem leaf powder. It helps address oily T-zone areas by regulating sebum production while simultaneously providing antibacterial benefits for acne-prone areas.

3. **Normal Skin**: Even individuals with normal skin can incorporate neem leaf powder into their skincare routine. It helps maintain the skin's natural balance, cleanse and purify the skin, and prevent the occurrence of acne and other skin issues.

4. **Sensitive Skin**: Neem leaf powder can be suitable for sensitive skin, but it's essential to use it with caution and in moderation. Some individuals with sensitive skin may find neem leaf powder too strong or irritating, so it's best to perform a patch test before using it on larger

areas of the skin. Diluting neem leaf powder with a gentle carrier like rose water or yogurt can help mitigate any potential sensitivity.

5. **Mature Skin**: While neem leaf powder is often associated with treating acne and oily skin, its antioxidant properties can benefit mature skin as well. The antioxidants help protect the skin from free radical damage, prevent premature aging, and promote a more youthful complexion.

Overall, neem leaf powder is versatile and can be beneficial for various skin types. However, it's essential to customize its usage based on individual skin concerns and sensitivities. If you experience any adverse reactions, such as excessive dryness or irritation, discontinue use and consult a dermatologist. Additionally, always follow up with a moisturizer after using neem leaf powder to prevent over-drying of the skin.

Benefits of neem leaf powder

Neem leaf powder, derived from the leaves of the neem tree (Azadirachta indica), is renowned for its numerous health and skincare benefits. Here are some of the key benefits of neem leaf powder:

1. **Antibacterial Properties**: Neem leaf powder contains compounds like nimbidin and nimbin, which exhibit strong antibacterial properties. It helps combat bacteria on the skin's surface, making it effective in treating acne and preventing future breakouts.

2. **Anti-inflammatory Effects**: Neem leaf powder possesses potent anti-inflammatory properties, which help reduce redness, swelling, and irritation. It is beneficial for soothing various skin conditions like eczema, psoriasis, and dermatitis.

3. **Antioxidant Activity**: The high antioxidant content in neem leaf powder helps protect the skin from damage caused by free radicals. Antioxidants help neutralize harmful molecules, preventing premature aging and promoting a more youthful complexion.

4. **Oil Control**: Neem leaf powder helps regulate sebum production, making it ideal for oily and acne-prone skin. It helps mattify the skin, reduce excess oiliness, and prevent clogged pores, blackheads, and acne breakouts.

5. **Skin Purification**: Neem leaf powder acts as a natural detoxifier, helping to purify and cleanse the skin by removing impurities, toxins, and bacteria. It helps maintain skin hygiene and prevents the buildup of harmful microbes.

6. **Skin Brightening**: Regular use of neem leaf powder can help lighten dark spots, hyperpigmentation, and blemishes, giving the skin a more even tone and brighter appearance. It also helps reduce the appearance of acne scars and post-inflammatory hyperpigmentation.

7. **Wound Healing**: Neem leaf powder promotes wound healing and tissue regeneration, making it beneficial for treating minor cuts, burns, and insect bites. It accelerates the healing process and reduces the risk of infection.

8. **Hair Care**: Neem leaf powder is also beneficial for hair health. It helps cleanse the scalp, remove excess oil and dandruff, and promote healthy hair growth. Neem leaf powder also has conditioning properties that add shine and softness to the hair.

9. **Oral Health**: Neem leaf powder can be used in oral care products like toothpaste and mouthwash due to its antibacterial properties. It helps prevent gum disease, tooth decay, and bad breath.

10. **Immune Support**: Consuming neem leaf powder or using it topically can help support the immune system and promote overall health and well-being.

These are just some of the many benefits of neem leaf powder. It is a versatile and potent ingredient that can be incorporated into various skincare, haircare, and health products to promote optimal health and vitality.

Side effects of neem leaf powder

While neem leaf powder offers numerous benefits for health and skincare, it's essential to be aware of potential side effects, especially when used in high concentrations or for prolonged periods. Here are some possible side effects of neem leaf powder:

1. **Skin Irritation**: Some individuals may experience skin irritation, redness, itching, or burning sensation when using neem leaf powder, especially if they have sensitive skin. This can occur due to the potent bioactive compounds present in neem.

2. **Dryness**: Neem leaf powder has astringent properties that can potentially dry out the skin, leading to excessive dryness or flakiness, particularly in individuals with already dry or sensitive skin.

3. **Allergic Reactions**: While rare, some people may be allergic to neem leaf powder or certain compounds present in it. Allergic reactions can manifest as skin rashes, hives, swelling, or difficulty breathing. If you have known allergies to plants in the mahogany family (Meliaceae), you may be at a higher risk of allergic reactions to neem.

4. **Photosensitivity**: Neem leaf powder may increase the skin's sensitivity to sunlight (photosensitivity) in some individuals, leading to a higher risk of sunburn or skin damage when exposed to UV radiation. It's important

to use sunscreen and limit sun exposure after applying neem leaf powder to the skin.

5. **Stomach Upset**: When consumed orally, neem leaf powder may cause stomach upset, nausea, vomiting, or diarrhea in some individuals, especially if taken in large doses. It's essential to use neem leaf powder in moderation and consult a healthcare professional before incorporating it into your diet.

6. **Liver Damage**: Prolonged or excessive consumption of neem leaf powder may potentially lead to liver damage in some individuals. Neem contains compounds that can be toxic to the liver if consumed in large quantities. It's crucial to use neem leaf powder responsibly and avoid overconsumption.

7. **Pregnancy and Breastfeeding**: There is limited research on the safety of neem leaf powder during pregnancy and breastfeeding. It's advisable for pregnant or breastfeeding women to avoid using neem leaf powder without consulting a healthcare professional.

8. **Drug Interactions**: Neem leaf powder may interact with certain medications, including antidiabetic drugs, immunosuppressants, and anticoagulants. If you are taking any medications, it's essential to consult a healthcare provider before using neem leaf powder to avoid potential interactions.

Overall, while neem leaf powder can offer numerous health and skincare benefits, it's essential to use it cautiously and be aware of potential side effects, especially if you have sensitive skin, allergies, or underlying health conditions. If you experience any adverse reactions, discontinue use, and consult a healthcare professional.

Different types of face pack can be prepared with neem leaf

powder.

Certainly! Neem leaf powder is a versatile ingredient that can be used to create various types of face packs suitable for different skin types and concerns. Here are a few DIY face pack recipes using neem leaf powder:

1. **Acne-Fighting Face Pack**:
   - Ingredients:
     - 1 tablespoon neem leaf powder
     - 1 tablespoon honey
     - 1 teaspoon turmeric powder
     - 1 teaspoon lemon juice
   - Instructions: Mix all the ingredients to form a smooth paste. Apply the pack to cleansed skin, focusing on acne-prone areas. Leave it on for 15-20 minutes, then rinse off with lukewarm water. This pack helps fight acne-causing bacteria, reduce inflammation, and fade acne scars.

2. **Oil-Control Face Pack**:
   - Ingredients:
     - 1 tablespoon neem leaf powder
     - 1 tablespoon yogurt
     - 1 teaspoon rose water.
   - Instructions: Mix the ingredients to form a paste. Apply it to the face, concentrating on oily areas. Leave it on for 15-20 minutes, then rinse off with water. This pack helps regulate sebum production, control excess oil, and prevent acne breakouts.

3. **Soothing Face Pack**:
   - Ingredients:
     - 1 tablespoon neem leaf powder

- 1 tablespoon aloe vera gel
- 1 teaspoon cucumber juice

- Instructions: Combine all the ingredients to make a smooth paste. Apply it to cleansed skin and leave it on for 15-20 minutes. Rinse off with water. This pack helps soothe irritated skin, reduce redness, and calm inflammation.

4. **Brightening Face Pack**:
   - Ingredients:
     - 1 tablespoon neem leaf powder
     - 1 tablespoon gram flour (besan)
     - 1 tablespoon raw milk

   - Instructions: Mix all the ingredients to form a paste. Apply the pack to the face and neck, leave it on for 15-20 minutes, then rinse off with water. This pack helps brighten the complexion, even out skin tone, and reduce pigmentation.

5. **Detoxifying Face Pack**:
   - Ingredients:
     - 1 tablespoon neem leaf powder
     - 1 tablespoon bentonite clay
     - 1 tablespoon apple cider vinegar

   - Instructions: Mix the ingredients to form a smooth paste. Apply it to the face, avoiding the eye area. Leave it on for 10-15 minutes, then rinse off with water. This pack helps detoxify the skin, draw out impurities, and unclog pores.

These are just a few examples of face packs you can create using neem leaf powder. Feel free to customize the recipes based on your skin type and specific concerns. Always perform a patch test before using any new skincare product and discontinue use if you

experience any irritation or allergic reactions.

Sandalwood Powder

Introduction to sandalwood powder

Sandalwood powder is a popular natural ingredient derived from the heartwood of the sandalwood tree (Santalum album). It has been used for centuries in Ayurvedic medicine and skincare rituals for its various benefits. Here are some of the properties and benefits of sandalwood powder:

1. **Antiseptic and Anti-inflammatory**: Sandalwood powder possesses antiseptic and anti-inflammatory properties, making it effective in soothing and calming irritated skin. It can help reduce redness, itching, and inflammation caused by conditions like acne, eczema, and rashes.

2. **Skin Brightening**: Sandalwood powder has skin-lightening properties that help fade dark spots, hyperpigmentation, and blemishes. Regular use of sandalwood powder can promote a more even skin tone and brighter complexion.

3. **Anti-aging**: Sandalwood powder contains antioxidants that help protect the skin from free radical damage, which can lead to premature aging. It helps reduce the appearance of fine lines, wrinkles, and other signs of aging, promoting smoother and younger-looking skin.

4. **Oil Control**: Sandalwood powder helps regulate sebum production, making it beneficial for oily and acne-prone skin. It helps mattify the skin, reduce shine, and prevent clogged pores and acne breakouts.

5. **Skin Soothing**: The cooling and soothing properties of sandalwood powder make it effective in relieving

sunburns, insect bites, and other skin irritations. It provides instant relief and comfort to the skin, making it feel refreshed and rejuvenated.

6. **Astringent**: Sandalwood powder has a mild astringent effect, which helps tighten and firm the skin, giving it a more toned appearance. It also helps minimize the appearance of pores and improve skin texture.

7. **Fragrance**: Sandalwood powder has a naturally pleasant aroma that is soothing and calming to the senses. It adds a luxurious scent to skincare products and can help relax the mind and body during skincare rituals.

8. **Hair Care**: Sandalwood powder is also beneficial for hair health. It helps cleanse the scalp, remove excess oil and dandruff, and promote healthy hair growth. Sandalwood powder also adds volume and shine to the hair.

Overall, sandalwood powder is a versatile and beneficial skincare ingredient with numerous uses and benefits for the skin and hair. It can be used in various DIY beauty treatments, including face masks, scrubs, and hair masks, to enhance the health and appearance of the skin and hair.

Sandalwood powder suitable for which skin type

Sandalwood powder is suitable for various skin types due to its gentle and versatile nature. Here's how it can benefit different skin types:

1. **Dry Skin**: Sandalwood powder is moisturizing and soothing, making it suitable for dry skin types. It helps hydrate the skin, relieve itching and irritation, and promote a soft and supple complexion.

2. **Oily Skin**: Sandalwood powder has astringent properties that help regulate sebum production, making

it beneficial for oily and acne-prone skin. It helps control excess oil, reduce shine, and prevent clogged pores and acne breakouts.

3. **Combination Skin**: Individuals with combination skin, where some areas of the face are oily while others are dry, can also benefit from sandalwood powder. It helps balance oil production in the T-zone while providing hydration and soothing properties to dry areas.

4. **Sensitive Skin**: Sandalwood powder is gentle and non-irritating, making it suitable for sensitive skin types. It helps calm inflammation, reduce redness, and soothe irritated skin without causing further sensitivity or allergic reactions.

5. **Mature Skin**: Sandalwood powder is rich in antioxidants, which help protect the skin from free radical damage and prevent premature aging. It helps reduce the appearance of fine lines, wrinkles, and age spots, promoting a more youthful and radiant complexion.

Overall, sandalwood powder is a versatile skincare ingredient that can benefit various skin types. Whether you have dry, oily, combination, sensitive, or mature skin, incorporating sandalwood powder into your skincare routine can help improve the health and appearance of your skin. However, it's essential to perform a patch test before using any new skincare product, including sandalwood powder, to ensure compatibility and minimize the risk of irritation or allergic reactions.

Benefits of sandalwood powder

Sandalwood powder, derived from the heartwood of the sandalwood tree (Santalum album), offers numerous benefits for skin, hair, and overall well-being. Here are some of the key benefits of sandalwood powder:

1. **Anti-inflammatory**: Sandalwood powder possesses anti-inflammatory properties that help reduce redness, swelling, and irritation on the skin. It can soothe various skin conditions, including acne, eczema, and sunburn.

2. **Antiseptic and Antimicrobial**: Sandalwood powder has natural antiseptic and antimicrobial properties, making it effective in preventing bacterial and fungal infections on the skin. It can help cleanse wounds, cuts, and insect bites, promoting faster healing.

3. **Skin Brightening**: Sandalwood powder contains compounds that help lighten and brighten the skin. Regular use can fade dark spots, hyperpigmentation, and blemishes, resulting in a more even skin tone and radiant complexion.

4. **Oil Control**: Sandalwood powder helps regulate sebum production, making it beneficial for oily and acne-prone skin. It helps control excess oil, reduce shine, and prevent clogged pores and acne breakouts.

5. **Astringent**: Sandalwood powder has mild astringent properties that help tighten and tone the skin. It can minimize the appearance of pores, improve skin texture, and give the skin a smoother and firmer appearance.

6. **Anti-aging**: Sandalwood powder is rich in antioxidants that help protect the skin from free radical damage, which can lead to premature aging. It helps reduce the appearance of fine lines, wrinkles, and age spots, promoting a more youthful complexion.

7. **Fragrance**: Sandalwood powder has a naturally soothing and calming aroma that can help relax the mind and body. It is often used in aromatherapy and skincare products to promote feelings of well-being and relaxation.

8. **Hair Care**: Sandalwood powder is beneficial for hair

health as well. It helps cleanse the scalp, remove excess oil and dandruff, and promote healthy hair growth. Sandalwood powder also adds volume and shine to the hair.

9. **Spiritual and Emotional Benefits**: Sandalwood powder has been used in traditional practices for its spiritual and emotional benefits. It is believed to have grounding and cantering properties, helping to calm the mind, reduce stress, and enhance meditation and mindfulness practices.

Overall, sandalwood powder is a versatile and beneficial ingredient that can be incorporated into various skincare, haircare, and wellness routines. Whether used topically or in aromatherapy, sandalwood powder offers a range of benefits for both physical and emotional well-being.

Side effects of sandalwood powder

While sandalwood powder is generally considered safe for topical use, there are some potential side effects and precautions to be aware of:

1. **Skin Irritation**: Some individuals may experience skin irritation or allergic reactions when using sandalwood powder, especially if they have sensitive skin or allergies to certain plant-based substances. Symptoms may include redness, itching, burning, or rash. It's essential to perform a patch test on a small area of skin before using sandalwood powder more extensively.

2. **Dryness**: Sandalwood powder has astringent properties that can potentially dry out the skin, particularly if used in high concentrations or for prolonged periods. Individuals with dry or sensitive skin may experience increased dryness, flakiness, or discomfort. It's advisable to use sandalwood powder in moderation

and follow up with a moisturizer if needed.

3. **Photosensitivity**: There is some evidence to suggest that sandalwood oil, a concentrated form of sandalwood extract, may increase the skin's sensitivity to sunlight (photosensitivity) when applied topically. While the risk with sandalwood powder may be lower, it's still advisable to use sunscreen and limit sun exposure after applying sandalwood powder to the skin, especially if using it in combination with other photosensitizing ingredients.

4. **Eye Irritation**: Avoid getting sandalwood powder into the eyes, as it may cause irritation or discomfort. If contact occurs, rinse the eyes thoroughly with water and seek medical attention if irritation persists.

5. **Adverse Reactions**: In rare cases, individuals may experience adverse reactions to sandalwood powder, such as headaches, nausea, or respiratory issues. If you experience any unusual symptoms after using sandalwood powder, discontinue use and consult a healthcare professional.

6. **Pregnancy and Breastfeeding**: There is limited research on the safety of using sandalwood powder during pregnancy and breastfeeding. While topical use is generally considered safe, it's advisable to consult a healthcare provider before using sandalwood powder if you are pregnant, breastfeeding, or have any underlying health conditions.

7. **Quality and Purity**: Ensure that you are using high-quality, pure sandalwood powder from reputable sources. Some products may be adulterated or contain added ingredients that could cause adverse reactions.

Overall, while sandalwood powder is generally safe for topical use, it's essential to be aware of potential side effects and use it cautiously, especially if you have sensitive skin or underlying health conditions. If you experience any adverse reactions, discontinue use, and consult a healthcare professional.

Different types of face pack can be prepared with sandalwood powder.

Certainly! Sandalwood powder is a versatile ingredient that can be used to create various types of face packs suitable for different skin types and concerns. Here are a few DIY face pack recipes using sandalwood powder:

1. **Soothing Sandalwood Face Pack**:
   - Ingredients:
     - 1 tablespoon sandalwood powder
     - 1 tablespoon rose water
     - 1 teaspoon honey
   - Instructions: Mix all the ingredients to form a smooth paste. Apply the pack to cleansed skin and leave it on for 15-20 minutes. Rinse off with lukewarm water. This pack helps soothe irritated skin, reduce redness, and provide hydration.

2. **Acne-Fighting Sandalwood Face Pack**:
   - Ingredients:
     - 1 tablespoon sandalwood powder
     - 1 tablespoon turmeric powder
     - 1 tablespoon yogurt
   - Instructions: Mix all the ingredients to form a paste. Apply the pack to the face, focusing on acne-prone areas. Leave it on for 15-20 minutes, then rinse off with water. This pack helps reduce inflammation, control excess oil, and prevent acne breakouts.

3. **Brightening Sandalwood Face Pack**:
   - Ingredients:
     - 1 tablespoon sandalwood powder
     - 1 tablespoon lemon juice
     - 1 teaspoon honey
   - Instructions: Combine all the ingredients to make a smooth paste. Apply the pack to the face and neck, leave it on for 15-20 minutes, then rinse off with water. This pack helps lighten dark spots, hyperpigmentation, and blemishes, giving the skin a brighter complexion.

4. **Hydrating Sandalwood Face Pack**:
   - Ingredients:
     - 1 tablespoon sandalwood powder
     - 1 tablespoon mashed avocado
     - 1 teaspoon almond oil
   - Instructions: Mix all the ingredients to form a creamy paste. Apply the pack to cleansed skin and leave it on for 20-30 minutes. Rinse off with lukewarm water. This pack helps nourish and moisturize dry skin, leaving it soft and supple.

5. **Cooling Sandalwood Face Pack**:
   - Ingredients:
     - 1 tablespoon sandalwood powder
     - 1 tablespoon cucumber juice
     - 1 teaspoon aloe vera gel
   - Instructions: Mix the ingredients to form a paste. Apply it to the face and leave it on for 15-20 minutes. Rinse off with water. This pack helps cool and refresh the skin, reduce puffiness, and soothe sunburns or irritated

skin.

These are just a few examples of face packs you can create using sandalwood powder. Feel free to customize the recipes based on your skin type and specific concerns. Always perform a patch test before using any new skincare product and discontinue use if you experience any irritation or allergic reactions.

Beetroot Powder

Introduction to beetroot powder

Beetroot powder is a vibrant, naturally derived powder made from dried beetroot. It offers a range of health and skincare benefits due to its rich nutritional profile and natural pigments. Here are some of the benefits and uses of beetroot powder:

1. **Antioxidant Properties**: Beetroot powder is high in antioxidants such as battalions and anthocyanins, which help protect the body from oxidative stress and free radical damage. Antioxidants contribute to overall health and may help reduce the risk of chronic diseases.

2. **Anti-inflammatory**: The battalions found in beetroot powder have anti-inflammatory properties, which can help reduce inflammation in the body. This may benefit individuals with inflammatory conditions such as arthritis or inflammatory skin conditions.

3. **Heart Health**: Beetroot powder contains nitrates, which are converted into nitric oxide in the body. Nitric oxide helps dilate blood vessels, improve blood flow, and lower blood pressure. Regular consumption of beetroot powder may support heart health and reduce the risk of cardiovascular diseases.

4. **Exercise Performance**: Some research suggests that the nitrates in beetroot powder may improve exercise performance and endurance by enhancing oxygen delivery to muscles. Athletes and fitness enthusiasts may benefit from incorporating beetroot powder into their pre-workout routine.

5. **Digestive Health**: Beetroot powder is rich in dietary fiber, which supports digestive health by promoting regular bowel movements and preventing constipation. Fiber also feeds beneficial gut bacteria, supporting a healthy gut microbiome.

6. **Skin Health**: Beetroot powder's antioxidant properties may benefit the skin by protecting against environmental damage and promoting a healthy

complexion. Some skincare products contain beetroot extract for its potential anti-aging and skin-brightening effects.

7. **Natural Food Colouring**: Beetroot powder is often used as a natural food colouring agent in various culinary applications. It adds a vibrant pink or red hue to foods and beverages without the need for artificial dyes.

8. **Detoxification**: Beetroot powder contains compounds that support liver function and detoxification processes in the body. Consuming beetroot powder may help support the body's natural detoxification pathways.

9. **Nutrient-Rich**: Beetroot powder is a good source of essential nutrients such as vitamins, minerals, and phytonutrients. It contains vitamins A, C, and K, folate, potassium, magnesium, and iron, among others, making it a nutritious addition to the diet.

10. **Weight Management**: Some studies suggest that beetroot powder may aid in weight management by promoting feelings of fullness, reducing appetite, and supporting metabolic health.

Overall, beetroot powder is a versatile ingredient that can be incorporated into a variety of recipes and products to promote health and well-being. However, individuals with certain health conditions, such as kidney stones or iron overload disorders, should consult with a healthcare professional before adding beetroot powder to their diet.

Beetroot powder suitable for which skin type

Beetroot powder can be beneficial for various skin types due to its antioxidant-rich and anti-inflammatory properties. Here's how it can suit different skin types:

1. **Normal Skin**: Individuals with normal skin can benefit

from the antioxidant properties of beetroot powder, which help protect the skin from environmental damage and premature aging. It can help maintain the skin's health and radiance.

2. **Dry Skin**: Beetroot powder is hydrating and nourishing, making it suitable for dry skin types. It helps moisturize the skin, improve hydration levels, and prevent dryness and flakiness. Beetroot powder may also enhance the skin's natural barrier function, reducing moisture loss.

3. **Oily Skin**: Despite its moisturizing properties, beetroot powder is lightweight and non-greasy, making it suitable for oily skin types. It helps hydrate the skin without clogging pores or adding excess oil. The antioxidant and anti-inflammatory properties of beetroot powder may also help reduce inflammation and balance sebum production in oily skin.

4. **Combination Skin**: Individuals with combination skin, where some areas are oily while others are dry, can benefit from the balancing properties of beetroot powder. It helps hydrate dry patches while regulating oil production in oily areas, promoting a more balanced complexion.

5. **Sensitive Skin**: Beetroot powder is generally gentle and well-tolerated, making it suitable for sensitive skin types. Its natural soothing and anti-inflammatory properties help calm irritation, redness, and inflammation, making it beneficial for sensitive or reactive skin.

6. **Aging Skin**: Beetroot powder's antioxidant properties help protect the skin from free radical damage, which can accelerate the aging process. It helps reduce the appearance of fine lines, wrinkles, and age spots, promoting a more youthful and radiant complexion.

Overall, beetroot powder is versatile and can benefit various skin types by promoting hydration, protecting against environmental damage, and reducing inflammation. Whether you have normal, dry, oily, combination, sensitive, or aging skin, incorporating beetroot powder into your skincare routine can help improve the health and appearance of your skin. However, it's essential to perform a patch test before using any new skincare product, including beetroot powder, to ensure compatibility and minimize the risk of irritation or allergic reactions.

Benefits of beetroot powder

Beetroot powder, made from dried and ground beetroot, offers numerous health benefits due to its rich nutritional profile and bioactive compounds. Here are some of the key benefits of beetroot powder:

1. **Rich in Antioxidants**: Beetroot powder is a potent source of antioxidants, including battalions, flavonoids, and vitamin C. Antioxidants help protect cells from oxidative stress caused by free radicals, reducing the risk of chronic diseases and promoting overall health.

2. **Heart Health**: The nitrates found in beetroot powder are converted into nitric oxide in the body, which helps dilate blood vessels, improve blood flow, and lower blood pressure. Regular consumption of beetroot powder may support cardiovascular health and reduce the risk of heart disease.

3. **Exercise Performance**: Beetroot powder may enhance exercise performance and endurance due to its nitrate content. Nitric oxide improves oxygen delivery to muscles, reducing fatigue and enhancing exercise efficiency. Athletes and fitness enthusiasts often use beetroot powder as a natural pre-workout supplement.

4. **Anti-inflammatory Properties**: The battalions in

beetroot powder have anti-inflammatory properties that help reduce inflammation in the body. Chronic inflammation is linked to various health conditions, including arthritis, diabetes, and heart disease. Beetroot powder may help alleviate inflammation and associated symptoms.

5. **Digestive Health**: Beetroot powder is rich in dietary fibre, which promotes digestive health by supporting regular bowel movements and preventing constipation. Fiber also feeds beneficial gut bacteria, promoting a healthy gut microbiome and overall digestive function.

6. **Detoxification**: Beetroot powder supports liver function and detoxification processes in the body. It helps eliminate toxins and waste products from the liver, kidneys, and other organs, supporting overall detoxification and cleansing.

7. **Blood Sugar Control**: Some studies suggest that beetroot powder may help regulate blood sugar levels and improve insulin sensitivity. The fibre and antioxidants in beetroot powder may help stabilize blood sugar levels and reduce the risk of diabetes-related complications.

8. **Weight Management**: Beetroot powder is low in calories and fat but high in fibre, making it a satisfying addition to a weight loss or weight management plan. The fibre content helps promote feelings of fullness, reduce appetite, and support healthy weight loss.

9. **Skin Health**: Beetroot powder's antioxidant and anti-inflammatory properties may benefit the skin by protecting against environmental damage, reducing inflammation, and promoting a healthy complexion. Some skincare products contain beetroot extract for its potential anti-aging and skin-brightening effects.

10. **Nutrient-Rich**: Beetroot powder is a good source of

essential nutrients such as vitamins, minerals, and phytonutrients. It contains vitamins A, C, and K, folate, potassium, magnesium, and iron, among others, making it a nutritious addition to the diet.

Overall, beetroot powder is a versatile and nutrient-rich superfood that offers numerous health benefits. Whether consumed as a dietary supplement, added to smoothies or recipes, or used in skincare products, beetroot powder can support overall health and well-being.

Side effects of beetroot powder

While beetroot powder is generally safe for most people when consumed in moderation, there are some potential side effects and considerations to be aware of:

1. **Beeturia**: Beeturia is a harmless condition characterized by the excretion of pink or red urine after consuming beetroot or beetroot products. This phenomenon occurs in some individuals due to the presence of betalain pigments in beets. Beeturia is not harmful and typically resolves on its own.

2. **Stomach Upset**: Some people may experience digestive discomfort, such as bloating, gas, or diarrhea, after consuming beetroot powder, particularly if they consume it in large amounts. This is often due to the high fibre content in beets, which can be difficult to digest for some individuals.

3. **Kidney Stones**: Beetroot powder is high in oxalates, compounds that can contribute to the formation of kidney stones in susceptible individuals. People with a history of kidney stones or those at risk of developing them may need to limit their intake of beetroot powder

or consult with a healthcare professional.

4. **Blood Pressure Changes**: While beetroot powder is known for its ability to lower blood pressure due to its nitrate content, consuming excessive amounts may lead to excessively low blood pressure (hypotension). Individuals taking blood pressure-lowering medications should use beetroot powder cautiously and monitor their blood pressure regularly.

5. **Allergic Reactions**: Some individuals may be allergic to components in beets, such as battalions or proteins. Allergic reactions to beetroot powder can manifest as itching, hives, swelling, or difficulty breathing. People with known allergies to beets or other plants in the Amaranthaceae family should avoid beetroot powder.

6. **Interactions with Medications**: Beetroot powder may interact with certain medications, including blood pressure-lowering drugs, medications for erectile dysfunction (such as sildenafil), and medications metabolized by the liver. If you are taking any medications, consult with a healthcare professional before using beetroot powder to avoid potential interactions.

7. **Blood Sugar Levels**: Beetroot powder may affect blood sugar levels, particularly in individuals with diabetes or those at risk of developing diabetes. While the fiber content in beetroot powder can help stabilize blood sugar levels, it's essential for people with diabetes to monitor their blood sugar closely when consuming beetroot powder.

8. **Risk of Gout**: Beetroot powder contains moderate levels of purines, which can increase uric acid levels in the body. People with gout or a history of gout should consume beetroot powder in moderation to avoid

exacerbating symptoms.

Overall, while beetroot powder offers numerous health benefits, it's essential to use it in moderation and be mindful of potential side effects, particularly if you have underlying health conditions or are taking medications. If you experience any adverse reactions after consuming beetroot powder, discontinue use and consult with a healthcare professional.

Different types of face pack can be prepared with beetroot powder.

Certainly! Beetroot powder can be used in various DIY face pack recipes to promote healthy and radiant skin. Here are a few different types of face packs that you can prepare using beetroot powder:

1. **Brightening Beetroot Face Pack:**
   - Ingredients:
     - 1 tablespoon beetroot powder
     - 1 tablespoon yogurt
     - 1 teaspoon honey
   - Instructions: Mix all the ingredients in a bowl to form a smooth paste. Apply the pack to cleansed skin and leave it on for 15-20 minutes. Rinse off with lukewarm water. This pack helps brighten the complexion, reduce dullness, and improve skin tone.

2. **Hydrating Beetroot Face Pack:**
   - Ingredients:
     - 1 tablespoon beetroot powder
     - 1 tablespoon mashed avocado
     - 1 teaspoon almond oil
   - Instructions: Combine all the ingredients to form a creamy paste. Apply the pack to the face

and leave it on for 20-30 minutes. Rinse off with lukewarm water. This pack helps nourish and moisturize dry skin, leaving it soft and hydrated.

3. **Cleansing Beetroot Face Pack**:
   - Ingredients:
     - 1 tablespoon beetroot powder
     - 1 tablespoon bentonite clay
     - 1 tablespoon rose water.
   - Instructions: Mix the ingredients to form a smooth paste. Apply the pack to the face, avoiding the eye area. Leave it on for 10-15 minutes, then rinse off with water. This pack helps cleanse the skin, remove impurities, and unclog pores.

4. **Anti-Aging Beetroot Face Pack**:
   - Ingredients:
     - 1 tablespoon beetroot powder
     - 1 tablespoon aloe vera gel
     - 1 teaspoon rosehip oil
   - Instructions: Combine all the ingredients to form a paste. Apply the pack to the face and neck, leave it on for 15-20 minutes, then rinse off with water. This pack helps reduce the appearance of fine lines, wrinkles, and age spots, promoting a more youthful complexion.

5. **Soothing Beetroot Face Pack**:
   - Ingredients:
     - 1 tablespoon beetroot powder
     - 1 tablespoon cucumber juice
     - 1 teaspoon oatmeal (optional)
   - Instructions: Mix all the ingredients to form a

paste. Apply it to the face and leave it on for 15-20 minutes. Rinse off with water. This pack helps soothe irritated skin, reduce redness, and calm inflammation.

These are just a few examples of face packs you can create using beetroot powder. Feel free to customize the recipes based on your skin type and specific concerns. Always perform a patch test before using any new skincare product, including beetroot powder, to ensure compatibility and minimize the risk of irritation or allergic reactions.

Turmeric Powder

Introduction to turmeric powder

Turmeric powder, derived from the root of the Curcuma longa plant, is a versatile spice known for its numerous health and skincare benefits. Here are some of the benefits and uses of turmeric powder:

1. **Anti-inflammatory Properties**: Turmeric contains curcumin, a compound known for its potent anti-inflammatory effects. It helps reduce inflammation in the body, alleviating symptoms of inflammatory conditions such as arthritis, asthma, and inflammatory bowel disease.

2. **Antioxidant Benefits**: Curcumin in turmeric acts as a powerful antioxidant, scavenging free radicals and protecting cells from oxidative damage. Antioxidants help prevent chronic diseases, slow down the aging process, and support overall health and well-being.

3. **Skin Health**: Turmeric has been used for centuries in traditional skincare remedies for its antimicrobial and anti-inflammatory properties. It can help soothe irritated skin, reduce acne, lighten dark spots and hyperpigmentation, and promote a clear and radiant complexion.

4. **Wound Healing**: Turmeric has natural antiseptic and antibacterial properties that promote wound healing and prevent infections. Applying turmeric paste to minor cuts, scrapes, and burns can help accelerate the healing process and reduce the risk of scarring.

5. **Digestive Health**: Turmeric aids digestion and promotes gastrointestinal health. It stimulates the production of bile, which helps break down fats and improve digestion. Turmeric may also alleviate symptoms of indigestion, bloating, and gas.

6. **Anti-cancer Properties**: Curcumin in turmeric has been studied for its potential anti-cancer properties. It may help prevent cancer development, inhibit the growth of cancer cells, and reduce the spread of tumours. However, more research is needed to confirm these effects.

7. **Joint Health**: Turmeric's anti-inflammatory properties may benefit individuals with joint pain and arthritis. It helps reduce pain, swelling, and stiffness in the joints, improving mobility and overall joint health.

8. **Brain Health**: Curcumin has neuroprotective properties that may help prevent neurodegenerative diseases such as Alzheimer's and Parkinson's disease. It enhances

brain function, promotes the growth of new neurons, and protects against age-related cognitive decline.

9. **Heart Health**: Turmeric supports cardiovascular health by reducing inflammation, improving blood circulation, and lowering cholesterol levels. It may help prevent heart disease, stroke, and other cardiovascular conditions.

10. **Immune Support**: Turmeric boosts the immune system and enhances immune function, helping the body fight off infections and illnesses more effectively.

Overall, turmeric powder is a potent and versatile spice with numerous health benefits. Whether consumed as a dietary supplement, used in cooking, or applied topically to the skin, turmeric can contribute to overall health and well-being. However, it's essential to use turmeric in moderation and consult with a healthcare professional if you have any underlying health conditions or are taking medications.

Turmeric powder suitable for which skin type

Turmeric powder can be suitable for various skin types, but its benefits may vary depending on individual skin concerns. Here's how turmeric powder can benefit different skin types:

1. **Normal Skin**: Turmeric powder can be beneficial for normal skin types as it helps promote a healthy complexion, reduce inflammation, and protect against environmental damage. It can help maintain skin balance and radiance.

2. **Dry Skin**: Turmeric powder has moisturizing and hydrating properties, making it suitable for dry skin types. It helps soothe dryness, improve skin elasticity, and promote a soft and supple complexion. Turmeric can be combined with moisturizing ingredients like yogurt or honey for added hydration.

3. **Oily Skin**: Turmeric powder is beneficial for oily skin types due to its anti-inflammatory and antimicrobial properties. It helps control excess oil production, reduce acne and breakouts, and minimize the appearance of pores. Turmeric can be combined with ingredients like yogurt or lemon juice for oil-balancing benefits.

4. **Combination Skin**: Individuals with combination skin can also benefit from turmeric powder. It helps balance oil production in the T-zone while providing hydration and soothing properties to dry areas. Combination skin types can use turmeric in face masks with ingredients that address both oily and dry skin concerns.

5. **Sensitive Skin**: Turmeric powder may be suitable for sensitive skin types, but it's essential to use it cautiously and perform a patch test first. Some individuals with sensitive skin may experience irritation or allergic reactions to turmeric. However, many people find that turmeric's anti-inflammatory properties help calm sensitive skin and reduce redness and irritation.

6. **Acne-Prone Skin**: Turmeric powder is known for its anti-inflammatory and antibacterial properties, making it beneficial for acne-prone skin. It helps reduce inflammation, unclog pores, and inhibit the growth of acne-causing bacteria. Turmeric can be combined with ingredients like honey, yogurt, or tea tree oil for acne-fighting benefits.

Overall, turmeric powder can be suitable for various skin types, but it's essential to consider individual skin concerns and sensitivities when using it. If you have specific skin issues or concerns, consult with a dermatologist or skincare professional before incorporating turmeric powder into your skincare routine. Additionally, perform a patch test before using any new skincare product containing turmeric to ensure compatibility and minimize the risk of irritation or allergic reactions.

Benefits of turmeric powder

Turmeric powder, derived from the root of the Curcuma longa plant, offers a wide range of health benefits due to its active compound, curcumin, and other bioactive components. Here are some of the key benefits of turmeric powder:

1. **Powerful Anti-inflammatory Properties**: Curcumin, the main active ingredient in turmeric, is known for its potent anti-inflammatory effects. It helps reduce inflammation in the body, alleviating symptoms of inflammatory conditions such as arthritis, asthma, and inflammatory bowel disease.

2. **Antioxidant Benefits**: Turmeric powder contains powerful antioxidants that help neutralize free radicals and protect cells from oxidative damage. Antioxidants play a crucial role in preventing chronic diseases, slowing down the aging process, and supporting overall health and well-being.

3. **Promotes Heart Health**: Curcumin in turmeric helps improve heart health by reducing inflammation, improving blood circulation, and lowering cholesterol levels. It may help prevent heart disease, stroke, and other cardiovascular conditions.

4. **Supports Digestive Health**: Turmeric aids digestion and promotes gastrointestinal health. It stimulates the production of bile, which helps break down fats and improve digestion. Turmeric may also alleviate symptoms of indigestion, bloating, and gas.

5. **Joint Health**: Turmeric's anti-inflammatory properties may benefit individuals with joint pain and arthritis. It helps reduce pain, swelling, and stiffness in the joints, improving mobility and overall joint health.

6. **Boosts Immune System**: Curcumin has immune-

boosting properties that help strengthen the immune system and enhance immune function. It helps the body fight off infections and illnesses more effectively.

7. **Supports Brain Health**: Curcumin has neuroprotective properties that may help prevent neurodegenerative diseases such as Alzheimer's and Parkinson's disease. It enhances brain function, promotes the growth of new neurons, and protects against age-related cognitive decline.

8. **Skin Health**: Turmeric has been used for centuries in traditional skincare remedies for its antimicrobial and anti-inflammatory properties. It can help soothe irritated skin, reduce acne, lighten dark spots and hyperpigmentation, and promote a clear and radiant complexion.

9. **Anti-cancer Properties**: Curcumin in turmeric has been studied for its potential anti-cancer properties. It may help prevent cancer development, inhibit the growth of cancer cells, and reduce the spread of tumours. However, more research is needed to confirm these effects.

10. **Liver Health**: Turmeric supports liver function and detoxification processes in the body. It helps eliminate toxins and waste products from the liver, supporting overall detoxification and cleansing.

Overall, turmeric powder is a potent and versatile spice with numerous health benefits. Whether consumed as a dietary supplement, used in cooking, or applied topically to the skin, turmeric can contribute to overall health and well-being. However, it's essential to use turmeric in moderation and consult with a healthcare professional if you have any underlying health conditions or are taking medications.

Side effects of turmeric powder

While turmeric powder is generally considered safe for most people when consumed in moderate amounts, excessive intake may cause side effects in some individuals. Here are some potential side effects and considerations associated with turmeric powder:

1. **Gastrointestinal Issues**: Consuming large amounts of turmeric powder may cause gastrointestinal issues such as nausea, vomiting, bloating, or diarrhea. Some people may be more sensitive to the effects of turmeric on the digestive system, especially if they have existing gastrointestinal conditions such as gastroesophageal reflux disease (GERD) or irritable bowel syndrome (IBS).

2. **Risk of Kidney Stones**: Turmeric contains oxalates, compounds that can contribute to the formation of kidney stones in susceptible individuals. People with a history of kidney stones or those at risk of developing them may need to limit their intake of turmeric powder.

3. **Increased Bleeding Risk**: Turmeric has blood-thinning properties and may increase the risk of bleeding, especially when consumed in large amounts or taken in supplement form. People who are taking blood-thinning medications such as warfarin or aspirin should use turmeric with caution and consult with a healthcare professional before incorporating it into their diet.

4. **Gallbladder Issues**: Turmeric may stimulate the production of bile, which could exacerbate gallbladder problems or cause gallbladder contractions in people with gallbladder disease. Individuals with gallbladder issues should use turmeric cautiously and consult with a healthcare provider.

5. **Allergic Reactions**: Some people may be allergic to turmeric or develop allergic reactions after consuming it. Allergic reactions to turmeric can manifest as

itching, hives, swelling, or difficulty breathing. People with known allergies to turmeric or other plants in the Zingiberaceae family (such as ginger) should avoid turmeric powder.

6. **Interactions with Medications**: Turmeric may interact with certain medications, including blood-thinning drugs, medications for diabetes, medications that reduce stomach acid (such as proton pump inhibitors), and drugs metabolized by the liver. If you are taking any medications, consult with a healthcare professional before using turmeric powder to avoid potential interactions.

7. **Pregnancy and Breastfeeding**: While turmeric is considered safe in culinary amounts, pregnant and breastfeeding women should avoid consuming large amounts of turmeric supplements or extracts due to limited safety data. High doses of turmeric may stimulate the uterus or cause gastrointestinal discomfort in some individuals.

8. **Yellow Staining**: Turmeric powder has strong pigments that can stain surfaces, clothing, and skin. Be cautious when handling turmeric powder and avoid contact with porous materials to prevent staining.

Overall, while turmeric powder offers numerous health benefits, it's essential to use it in moderation and be mindful of potential side effects, especially in certain populations or when consumed in large amounts. If you experience any adverse reactions after consuming turmeric powder, discontinue use and consult with a healthcare professional.

Different types of face pack can be prepared with turmeric powder.

Turmeric powder is a versatile ingredient that can be used in various DIY face pack recipes to address different skin concerns. Here are some types of face packs you can prepare using turmeric powder:

1. **Brightening Turmeric Face Pack**:
    - Ingredients:
        - 1 tablespoon turmeric powder
        - 1 tablespoon yogurt
        - 1 teaspoon honey
    - Instructions: Mix all the ingredients in a bowl to form a smooth paste. Apply the pack to cleansed skin and leave it on for 15-20 minutes. Rinse off with lukewarm water. This pack helps brighten the complexion, reduce dullness, and improve skin tone.

2. **Acne-Fighting Turmeric Face Pack**:
    - Ingredients:
        - 1 tablespoon turmeric powder
        - 1 tablespoon chickpea flour (besan)
        - 1 tablespoon rose water.
    - Instructions: Combine all the ingredients to form a paste. Apply the pack to the face, focusing on acne-prone areas. Leave it on for 15-20 minutes, then rinse off with water. This pack helps reduce acne, control excess oil, and soothe inflammation.

3. **Hydrating Turmeric Face Pack**:
    - Ingredients:
        - 1 tablespoon turmeric powder
        - 1 tablespoon mashed avocado
        - 1 teaspoon almond oil
    - Instructions: Mix all the ingredients to form a creamy paste. Apply the pack to the face

and leave it on for 20-30 minutes. Rinse off with lukewarm water. This pack helps nourish and moisturize dry skin, leaving it soft and hydrated.

4. **Anti-inflammatory Turmeric Face Pack**:
   - Ingredients:
     - 1 tablespoon turmeric powder
     - 1 tablespoon aloe vera gel
     - 1 teaspoon coconut oil
   - Instructions: Combine all the ingredients to form a paste. Apply it to the face and leave it on for 15-20 minutes. Rinse off with water. This pack helps soothe irritated skin, reduce redness, and calm inflammation.

5. **Exfoliating Turmeric Face Pack**:
   - Ingredients:
     - 1 tablespoon turmeric powder
     - 1 tablespoon oatmeal
     - 1 tablespoon honey
   - Instructions: Mix the ingredients to form a paste. Gently massage the pack onto damp skin using circular motions for 1-2 minutes, then leave it on for an additional 10-15 minutes. Rinse off with water. This pack helps exfoliate dead skin cells, unclog pores, and reveal smoother skin.

6. **Anti-aging Turmeric Face Pack**:
   - Ingredients:
     - 1 tablespoon turmeric powder
     - 1 tablespoon yogurt
     - 1 teaspoon rosehip oil
   - Instructions: Mix all the ingredients to form a

paste. Apply the pack to the face and neck, leave it on for 15-20 minutes, then rinse off with water. This pack helps reduce the appearance of fine lines, wrinkles, and age spots, promoting a more youthful complexion.

These are just a few examples of face packs you can create using turmeric powder. Feel free to customize the recipes based on your skin type and specific concerns. Always perform a patch test before using any new skincare product containing turmeric to ensure compatibility and minimize the risk of irritation or allergic reactions.

Besan Powder

Introduction to besan powder

Besan powder, also known as gram flour or chickpea flour, is a versatile ingredient that offers various benefits for skincare. Here are some of the benefits of besan powder:

1. **Cleanses the Skin**: Besan powder has natural cleansing properties that help remove dirt, oil, and impurities from the skin. It acts as a gentle exfoliant, removing dead skin cells and unclogging pores, leaving the skin clean and refreshed.

2. **Controls Oiliness**: Besan powder can help regulate sebum production, making it beneficial for oily and acne-prone skin. It absorbs excess oil from the skin's surface without stripping away essential moisture, helping to mattify the complexion and prevent breakouts.

3. **Exfoliates the Skin**: The slightly coarse texture of besan powder makes it an excellent natural exfoliant. Regular exfoliation with besan powder helps slough off dead skin cells, promoting cell turnover and revealing smoother, brighter skin underneath.

4. **Lightens Dark Spots**: Besan powder contains natural enzymes that can help lighten dark spots, hyperpigmentation, and acne scars over time. Regular use of besan powder in skincare routines can help even out the skin tone and fade discoloration.

5. **Soothes Irritation**: Besan powder has soothing properties that can help calm irritated or inflamed skin. It can be particularly beneficial for individuals with sensitive skin, eczema, or rosacea, as it helps reduce redness and inflammation.

6. **Treats Acne**: Besan powder has antimicrobial properties that make it effective in combating acne-causing bacteria. When used regularly as part of a skincare routine, besan powder can help prevent and reduce acne breakouts, resulting in clearer skin.

7. **Nourishes the Skin**: Besan powder contains vitamins and minerals that nourish the skin, including vitamin B6, zinc, and magnesium. These nutrients help promote skin health, improve elasticity, and maintain a youthful appearance.

8. **Reduces Facial Hair Growth**: Regular application of besan powder with other ingredients like turmeric and yogurt can help weaken hair follicles and inhibit facial hair growth over time. This natural remedy is often used as an alternative to harsh chemical hair removal methods.

9. **Brightens the Complexion**: Besan powder has skin-brightening properties that help impart a natural glow to the complexion. It helps remove dullness and fatigue from the skin, leaving it looking radiant and refreshed.

10. **Tightens Pores**: Besan powder has a mild astringent effect that helps tighten and minimize the appearance of pores. Regular use of besan powder in skincare

routines can help refine the skin's texture and reduce the visibility of enlarged pores.

Overall, besan powder is a versatile skincare ingredient that offers a wide range of benefits for various skin types. Whether used alone or in combination with other natural ingredients, besan powder can help improve the overall health and appearance of the skin.

Besan powder suitable for which skin type

Besan powder, also known as gram flour or chickpea flour, is suitable for various skin types due to its gentle and versatile nature. Here's how besan powder can benefit different skin types:

1. **Normal Skin**: Besan powder is generally well-tolerated by normal skin types. It helps cleanse the skin, remove impurities, and maintain its natural balance without stripping away essential moisture. Besan powder can leave normal skin feeling clean, refreshed, and rejuvenated.

2. **Dry Skin**: While besan powder can be slightly drying, especially when used alone, it can still be beneficial for dry skin types when combined with hydrating ingredients such as yogurt, honey, or milk. These additions help moisturize the skin while reaping the benefits of besan powder's exfoliating and cleansing properties.

3. **Oily Skin**: Besan powder is particularly beneficial for oily skin types as it helps absorb excess oil, unclog pores, and regulate sebum production. It acts as a natural cleanser and exfoliant, leaving the skin feeling fresh, matte, and less prone to breakouts. Using besan powder in face masks or cleansers can help control oiliness and promote a clearer complexion.

4. **Combination Skin**: Individuals with combination skin

can also benefit from besan powder by customizing their skincare routine to address specific concerns in different areas of the face. For example, using besan powder-based masks on oily zones and incorporating moisturizing ingredients on dry areas can help balance combination skin and promote overall skin health.

5. **Sensitive Skin**: Besan powder is generally gentle and well-tolerated by sensitive skin types, but it's essential to be cautious and perform a patch test before using it extensively. Some individuals with sensitive skin may find besan powder irritating, especially when used alone or in combination with harsh ingredients. However, when combined with soothing ingredients such as yogurt, cucumber, or aloe vera, besan powder can help calm inflammation and reduce redness in sensitive skin.

Overall, besan powder is suitable for a wide range of skin types, but its effectiveness may vary depending on individual skin concerns and sensitivities. It's essential to customize skincare routines accordingly and experiment with different formulations to find what works best for your skin. If you have specific skin issues or concerns, consult with a dermatologist or skincare professional for personalized recommendations.

Benefits of besan powder

Besan powder, also known as gram flour or chickpea flour, offers numerous benefits for the skin due to its unique composition and properties. Here are some of the key benefits of besan powder for skincare:

1. **Exfoliation**: Besan powder has a slightly coarse texture, making it an excellent natural exfoliant. It helps remove dead skin cells, dirt, and impurities from the skin's surface, revealing smoother, brighter skin underneath.

2. **Oil Control**: Besan powder has natural oil-absorbing

properties that help control excess oil production on the skin. It mattifies the complexion, reduces shine, and helps prevent clogged pores, making it particularly beneficial for oily and acne-prone skin types.

3. **Cleansing**: Besan powder acts as a gentle cleanser, effectively removing dirt, makeup, and impurities from the skin without stripping away its natural oils. It helps maintain the skin's pH balance and keeps it clean and refreshed.

4. **Brightening**: Besan powder contains enzymes that help lighten dark spots, hyperpigmentation, and acne scars over time. Regular use of besan powder can help even out the skin tone and promote a brighter, more radiant complexion.

5. **Soothing**: Besan powder has soothing properties that help calm irritated or inflamed skin. It can help reduce redness, itching, and inflammation associated with conditions like acne, eczema, or rosacea.

6. **Tightening**: Besan powder has a mild astringent effect that helps tighten and firm the skin. It helps minimize the appearance of enlarged pores, refine the skin's texture, and improve overall skin tone and elasticity.

7. **Anti-acne**: Besan powder has antimicrobial properties that help fight acne-causing bacteria and prevent breakouts. It helps cleanse the pores, reduce inflammation, and promote clearer, healthier-looking skin.

8. **Moisturizing**: Besan powder can be combined with hydrating ingredients like yogurt, honey, or milk to create moisturizing face masks. These masks help hydrate and nourish the skin, leaving it soft, supple, and moisturized.

9. **Anti-aging**: Besan powder contains antioxidants that

help protect the skin from environmental damage and signs of aging. It helps reduce the appearance of fine lines, wrinkles, and age spots, promoting a more youthful complexion.

10. **Hair Removal**: Besan powder can be used as a natural hair removal remedy when mixed with other ingredients like turmeric and yogurt. It weakens hair follicles and inhibits hair growth over time, making it an alternative to harsh chemical hair removal methods.

Overall, besan powder is a versatile skincare ingredient that offers a wide range of benefits for various skin concerns. Whether used alone or in combination with other natural ingredients, besan powder can help improve the overall health and appearance of the skin.

Side effects of besan powder

While besan powder is generally safe for most people when used topically, some individuals may experience side effects or allergic reactions. Here are some potential side effects and considerations associated with besan powder:

1. **Skin Irritation**: Besan powder can be abrasive for some individuals, especially those with sensitive or easily irritated skin. Using besan powder in its raw form or in combination with harsh exfoliating ingredients may cause redness, irritation, or itching. It's essential to perform a patch test before applying besan powder to a larger area of the skin to assess sensitivity.

2. **Dryness**: Besan powder has natural absorbent properties that can help control oiliness, but excessive use or leaving it on the skin for too long may lead to over-drying. This can result in skin tightness, flakiness, or discomfort, especially for individuals with dry or dehydrated skin. It's important to balance the use of

besan powder with hydrating ingredients to prevent excessive dryness.

3. **Allergic Reactions**: Some individuals may be allergic to besan powder or develop allergic reactions after using it. Allergic reactions can manifest as itching, redness, swelling, hives, or rash. If you have known allergies to chickpeas or legumes, it's best to avoid using besan powder or perform a patch test before using it on the skin.

4. **Contact Dermatitis**: Prolonged or repeated exposure to besan powder may lead to contact dermatitis in susceptible individuals. Contact dermatitis is a condition characterized by inflammation, redness, and irritation of the skin. It can occur due to sensitivity to certain components in besan powder or due to abrasive friction during application.

5. **Skin Sensitivity**: Individuals with compromised skin barrier function or underlying skin conditions such as eczema, psoriasis, or rosacea may be more prone to experiencing side effects from besan powder. It's essential to consult with a dermatologist before incorporating besan powder into skincare routines, especially for those with pre-existing skin conditions.

6. **Inhalation Risks**: When using besan powder in DIY face masks or scrubs, there's a risk of inhaling fine particles, which may irritate the respiratory system, especially for individuals with asthma or allergies. It's important to use besan powder in a well-ventilated area and avoid breathing in excess dust.

Overall, while besan powder offers numerous benefits for skincare, it's essential to use it cautiously and be mindful of potential side effects, especially for individuals with sensitive skin or underlying skin conditions. If you experience any adverse reactions after using besan powder, discontinue use and consult with a dermatologist or healthcare professional for guidance.

Different types of face pack can be prepared with besan powder.

Certainly! Besan powder, also known as gram flour or chickpea flour, is a versatile ingredient that can be used to create a variety of DIY face packs suitable for different skin types and concerns. Here are some types of face packs you can prepare using besan powder:

1. **Brightening Face Pack**:
    - Ingredients:
        - 2 tablespoons besan powder
        - 1 tablespoon yogurt
        - 1 teaspoon honey
    - Instructions: Mix all the ingredients to form a smooth paste. Apply the pack to cleansed skin and leave it on for 15-20 minutes. Rinse off with lukewarm water. This pack helps brighten the complexion and improve skin tone.

2. **Acne-Fighting Face Pack**:
    - Ingredients:
        - 2 tablespoons besan powder
        - 1 tablespoon rose water.
        - 1 teaspoon turmeric powder
    - Instructions: Combine all the ingredients to form a paste. Apply the pack to the face, focusing on acne-prone areas. Leave it on for 15-20 minutes, then rinse off with water. This pack helps reduce acne and prevent breakouts.

3. **Hydrating Face Pack**:
    - Ingredients:
        - 2 tablespoons besan powder

- 1 tablespoon mashed avocado

- 1 teaspoon almond oil

- Instructions: Mix all the ingredients to form a creamy paste. Apply the pack to the face and leave it on for 20-30 minutes. Rinse off with lukewarm water. This pack helps moisturize and nourish dry skin.

4. **Exfoliating Face Pack:**
   - Ingredients:
     - 2 tablespoons besan powder

     - 1 tablespoon oatmeal

     - 1 tablespoon yogurt

   - Instructions: Mix the ingredients to form a paste. Gently massage the pack onto damp skin using circular motions for 1-2 minutes, then leave it on for an additional 10-15 minutes. Rinse off with water. This pack helps remove dead skin cells and reveal smoother skin.

5. **Soothing Face Pack:**
   - Ingredients:
     - 2 tablespoons besan powder

     - 1 tablespoon cucumber juice

     - 1 teaspoon aloe vera gel

   - Instructions: Combine all the ingredients to form a paste. Apply it to the face and leave it on for 15-20 minutes. Rinse off with water. This pack helps calm and soothe irritated skin.

6. **Oil-Control Face Pack:**
   - Ingredients:
     - 2 tablespoons besan powder

     - 1 tablespoon lemon juice

- 1 teaspoon rose water.

- Instructions: Mix all the ingredients to form a paste. Apply the pack to the face, focusing on oily areas. Leave it on for 15-20 minutes, then rinse off with water. This pack helps control excess oil and reduce shine.

These are just a few examples of face packs you can create using besan powder. Feel free to customize the recipes based on your skin type and specific concerns. Always perform a patch test before using any new skincare product containing besan powder to ensure compatibility and minimize the risk of irritation or allergic reactions.

Green Gram Powder

Introduction to green gram powder

Green gram powder, also known as mung bean powder or moong dal powder, is derived from ground mung beans and offers various benefits for skincare. Here are some of the benefits of green gram powder:

1. **Gentle Exfoliation**: Green gram powder has a fine texture, making it a gentle exfoliant suitable for sensitive skin types. It helps remove dead skin cells, dirt, and impurities from the skin's surface, leaving it smooth and refreshed.

2. **Cleansing**: Green gram powder acts as a natural cleanser, effectively removing dirt, oil, and makeup residues from the skin without stripping away its natural oils. It helps unclog pores and prevent acne breakouts, making it suitable for oily and acne-prone skin types.

3. **Soothing**: Green gram powder has soothing properties that help calm irritated or inflamed skin. It can help reduce redness, itching, and inflammation associated with conditions like eczema, rosacea, or sunburn.

4. **Oil Control**: Green gram powder helps absorb excess oil from the skin's surface, making it beneficial for individuals with oily or combination skin. It mattifies the complexion, reduces shine, and minimizes the appearance of enlarged pores.

5. **Brightening**: Green gram powder contains vitamins and minerals that help promote a brighter, more radiant complexion. Regular use of green gram powder can help fade dark spots, hyperpigmentation, and acne scars, resulting in a more even skin tone.

6. **Anti-aging**: Green gram powder contains antioxidants that help protect the skin from environmental damage and signs of aging. It helps reduce the appearance of fine lines, wrinkles, and age spots, promoting a more youthful complexion.

7. **Moisturizing**: Green gram powder can be combined with hydrating ingredients like yogurt, honey, or milk to create moisturizing face masks. These masks help hydrate and nourish the skin, leaving it soft, supple, and moisturized.

8. **Toning**: Green gram powder has astringent properties that help tone and tighten the skin. It helps minimize the appearance of pores, refine the skin's texture, and improve overall skin tone and elasticity.

Overall, green gram powder is a versatile skincare ingredient that offers a wide range of benefits for various skin types. Whether used alone or in combination with other natural ingredients, green gram powder can help improve the overall health and appearance of the skin.

Geen gram powder suitable for which skin type

Green gram powder, also known as mung bean powder or moong dal powder, is generally suitable for all skin types due to its gentle and nourishing properties. Here's how green gram powder can benefit different skin types:

1. **Normal Skin**: Green gram powder is gentle enough for normal skin types and can help maintain the skin's natural balance. It provides gentle exfoliation, removes impurities, and promotes a smooth and radiant complexion without causing dryness or irritation.

2. **Dry Skin**: Green gram powder is hydrating and moisturizing, making it suitable for dry skin types. It helps cleanse the skin without stripping away its natural oils and leaves it feeling soft, supple, and nourished. Combining green gram powder with moisturizing ingredients like yogurt, honey, or milk can enhance its hydrating properties.

3. **Oily Skin**: Green gram powder is beneficial for oily skin types as it helps absorb excess oil and unclog pores. It mattifies the complexion, reduces shine, and minimizes the risk of acne breakouts. Using green gram powder in face masks or cleansers can help control oiliness and promote a clearer, more balanced complexion.

4. **Combination Skin**: Individuals with combination skin can also benefit from green gram powder by customizing their skincare routine to address specific concerns in different areas of the face. For example, using green gram powder-based masks on oily zones and incorporating hydrating ingredients on dry areas can help balance combination skin and promote overall skin health.

5. **Sensitive Skin**: Green gram powder is gentle and soothing, making it suitable for sensitive skin types. It helps cleanse the skin without causing irritation or redness and can be used safely on delicate skin areas. However, it's essential to perform a patch

test before using green gram powder extensively to ensure compatibility and minimize the risk of allergic reactions.

Overall, green gram powder is versatile and well-tolerated by most skin types. However, individual reactions may vary, so it's essential to monitor your skin's response and adjust usage accordingly. If you have specific skin concerns or conditions, consult with a dermatologist or skincare professional for personalized recommendations.

Benefits of green gram powder

Green gram powder, also known as mung bean powder or moong dal powder, offers a variety of benefits for skin and hair care due to its natural properties and nutrient content. Here are some of the key benefits of green gram powder:

1. **Gentle Exfoliation**: Green gram powder has a fine texture, making it an excellent natural exfoliant. It helps remove dead skin cells, dirt, and impurities from the skin's surface, leaving it smooth and refreshed. Regular exfoliation with green gram powder promotes cell turnover and reveals brighter, healthier-looking skin.

2. **Cleansing**: Green gram powder acts as a gentle cleanser, effectively removing dirt, oil, and makeup residues from the skin without stripping away its natural oils. It helps unclog pores and prevent acne breakouts, making it suitable for oily and acne-prone skin types.

3. **Soothing**: Green gram powder has soothing properties that help calm irritated or inflamed skin. It can help reduce redness, itching, and inflammation associated with conditions like eczema, rosacea, or sunburn. Green gram powder can also be used to soothe insect bites and minor skin irritations.

4. **Oil Control**: Green gram powder helps absorb excess

oil from the skin's surface, making it beneficial for individuals with oily or combination skin. It mattifies the complexion, reduces shine, and minimizes the appearance of enlarged pores. Regular use of green gram powder helps balance oil production and promote a clearer, more balanced complexion.

5. **Brightening**: Green gram powder contains vitamins and minerals that help promote a brighter, more radiant complexion. Regular use of green gram powder can help fade dark spots, hyperpigmentation, and acne scars, resulting in a more even skin tone. It also helps improve skin texture and gives the skin a healthy glow.

6. **Moisturizing**: Green gram powder is hydrating and nourishing, making it suitable for dry and sensitive skin types. It helps retain moisture in the skin, leaving it soft, supple, and moisturized. Combining green gram powder with hydrating ingredients like yogurt, honey, or milk enhances its moisturizing properties.

7. **Hair Care**: Green gram powder can also benefit hair health by promoting stronger, healthier hair growth. It contains proteins and nutrients that nourish the hair follicles, prevent hair loss, and improve scalp health. Green gram powder can be used as a natural hair mask to condition the hair and scalp, reduce dandruff, and add shine to the hair.

Overall, green gram powder is a versatile ingredient that offers a wide range of benefits for skin and hair care. Whether used alone or in combination with other natural ingredients, green gram powder can help improve the overall health and appearance of the skin and hair.

Side effects of green gram powder

While green gram powder is generally safe for topical use, some individuals may experience side effects or allergic reactions. Here are some potential side effects and considerations associated with green gram powder:

1. **Skin Irritation**: Some people may experience skin irritation, redness, itching, or rash after using green gram powder. This could be due to sensitivity to certain components in the powder or excessive friction during application. It's essential to perform a patch test before using green gram powder extensively on the skin.

2. **Allergic Reactions**: Individuals with allergies to legumes or beans may be allergic to green gram powder. Allergic reactions can manifest as itching, swelling, hives, or difficulty breathing. If you have known allergies to legumes, it's best to avoid using green gram powder or consult with a healthcare professional before using it.

3. **Excessive Dryness**: Green gram powder can have a drying effect on the skin, especially when used alone or in combination with drying ingredients. Using green gram powder too frequently or leaving it on the skin for extended periods may lead to excessive dryness, tightness, or flakiness, particularly for individuals with dry or sensitive skin.

4. **Clogging of Drains**: When washing off green gram powder masks or scrubs, it's important to be cautious as the particles can accumulate and potentially clog drains or pipes if not properly rinsed away.

5. **Inhalation Risks**: When using green gram powder in DIY face masks or scrubs, there's a risk of inhaling fine particles, which may irritate the respiratory system, especially for individuals with asthma or allergies. It's important to use green gram powder in a well-ventilated area and avoid breathing in excess dust.

6. **Staining**: Green gram powder can potentially stain fabrics or surfaces, like other natural powders. Be cautious when applying green gram powder masks to avoid contact with clothing or porous materials.

7. **Eye Irritation**: Avoid getting green gram powder into the eyes, as it can cause irritation or discomfort. If accidental contact occurs, rinse thoroughly with water.

Overall, while green gram powder offers numerous benefits for skin and hair care, it's essential to use it cautiously and be mindful of potential side effects, especially for individuals with sensitive skin or allergies. If you experience any adverse reactions after using green gram powder, discontinue use and consult with a dermatologist or healthcare professional for further guidance.

Different types of face pack can be prepared with green gram powder.

Certainly! Green gram powder, also known as mung bean powder or moong dal powder, can be used to create a variety of DIY face packs suitable for different skin types and concerns. Here are some types of face packs you can prepare using green gram powder:

1. **Exfoliating Face Pack:**
   - Ingredients:
     - 2 tablespoons green gram powder
     - 1 tablespoon yogurt
     - 1 teaspoon honey
   - Instructions: Mix all the ingredients to form a paste. Gently massage onto damp skin in circular motions for 1-2 minutes, then leave it on for an additional 10-15 minutes. Rinse off with lukewarm water. This pack helps remove dead skin cells, unclog pores, and reveal smoother skin.

2. **Brightening Face Pack**:
   - Ingredients:
     - 2 tablespoons green gram powder
     - 1 tablespoon tomato juice
     - 1 teaspoon lemon juice
   - Instructions: Mix all the ingredients to form a paste. Apply the pack to the face and leave it on for 15-20 minutes. Rinse off with water. This pack helps lighten dark spots, improve skin tone, and brighten the complexion.

3. **Soothing Face Pack**:
   - Ingredients:
     - 2 tablespoons green gram powder
     - 1 tablespoon cucumber juice
     - 1 teaspoon aloe vera gel
   - Instructions: Mix all the ingredients to form a paste. Apply it to the face and leave it on for 15-20 minutes. Rinse off with water. This pack helps calm and soothe irritated or inflamed skin, reducing redness and inflammation.

4. **Oil-Control Face Pack**:
   - Ingredients:
     - 2 tablespoons green gram powder
     - 1 tablespoon rose water.
     - 1 teaspoon Multani Miti (fuller's earth)
   - Instructions: Mix all the ingredients to form a paste. Apply the pack to the face, focusing on oily areas. Leave it on for 15-20 minutes, then rinse off with water. This pack helps absorb excess oil, tighten pores, and control shine.

5. **Hydrating Face Pack**:
   - Ingredients:

- 2 tablespoons green gram powder

- 1 tablespoon mashed ripe banana.

- 1 teaspoon honey

- Instructions: Mix all the ingredients to form a paste. Apply the pack to the face and leave it on for 15-20 minutes. Rinse off with lukewarm water. This pack helps moisturize and nourish dry or dehydrated skin, leaving it soft and supple.

6. **Anti-Acne Face Pack**:
   - Ingredients:
     - 2 tablespoons green gram powder

     - 1 tablespoon neem powder

     - 1 teaspoon turmeric powder

     - Rose water (as needed for consistency)

   - Instructions: Mix all the ingredients to form a paste. Apply the pack to the face, focusing on acne-prone areas. Leave it on for 15-20 minutes, then rinse off with water. This pack helps reduce acne, control inflammation, and prevent breakouts.

These are just a few examples of face packs you can create using green gram powder. Feel free to customize the recipes based on your skin type and specific concerns. Always perform a patch test before using any new skincare product containing green gram powder to ensure compatibility and minimize the risk of irritation or allergic reactions.

<u>**Lemon Peel Powder**</u>

Introduction to lemon peel powder

Lemon peel powder is derived from dried lemon peels and is known for its various skincare benefits. Here are some of the benefits of lemon peel powder:

1. **Exfoliation**: Lemon peel powder has natural exfoliating properties due to its slightly coarse texture. It helps remove dead skin cells, dirt, and impurities from the skin's surface, revealing smoother and brighter skin underneath.

2. **Brightening**: Lemon peel powder contains citric acid, which helps lighten dark spots, hyperpigmentation, and

acne scars. Regular use of lemon peel powder can help even out the skin tone and promote a more radiant complexion.

3. **Cleansing**: Lemon peel powder acts as a natural cleanser, effectively removing excess oil, dirt, and makeup residues from the skin. It helps unclog pores and prevent acne breakouts, making it beneficial for oily and acne-prone skin types.

4. **Oil Control**: Lemon peel powder has astringent properties that help control excess oil production on the skin. It helps mattify the complexion, reduce shine, and minimize the appearance of enlarged pores.

5. **Antioxidant Protection**: Lemon peel powder contains antioxidants such as vitamin C, which help protect the skin from environmental damage caused by free radicals. It helps prevent premature aging signs such as fine lines, wrinkles, and sagging skin.

6. **Skin Lightening**: Lemon peel powder contains natural bleaching agents that help lighten skin pigmentation and discoloration. It can be used to brighten dark elbows, knees, and underarms, as well as to lighten suntan.

7. **Anti-inflammatory**: Lemon peel powder has anti-inflammatory properties that help soothe irritated or inflamed skin. It can help reduce redness, itching, and inflammation associated with acne, eczema, or sunburn.

8. **Refreshing**: Lemon peel powder has a refreshing and invigorating scent that uplifts the mood and rejuvenates the senses. It can be used in homemade skincare products like scrubs, masks, and bath salts for a spa-like experience.

9. **Natural Deodorizer**: Lemon peel powder has natural

deodorizing properties that help neutralize unpleasant Odors on the skin. It can be used in foot scrubs or body powders to keep the skin feeling fresh and Odor-free.

10. **Hair Care**: Lemon peel powder can also benefit hair health by promoting scalp health, reducing dandruff, and adding shine to the hair. It can be used in homemade hair masks or rinses to nourish and strengthen the hair strands.

Overall, lemon peel powder is a versatile ingredient that offers a wide range of benefits for skincare and hair care. Whether used alone or in combination with other natural ingredients, lemon peel powder can help improve the overall health and appearance of the skin and hair.

Lemon peel powder suitable for which skin type

Lemon peel powder is generally suitable for most skin types, but its use should be approached with caution, especially for individuals with sensitive or dry skin. Here's a breakdown of its suitability for different skin types:

1. **Oily Skin**: Lemon peel powder can be particularly beneficial for oily skin types due to its astringent properties. It helps control excess oil production, mattify the complexion, and reduce shine. The exfoliating action of lemon peel powder also helps unclog pores, preventing acne breakouts and blackheads.

2. **Combination Skin**: Individuals with combination skin can also benefit from lemon peel powder, but they should be mindful of potential dryness in drier areas of the face. Using lemon peel powder in moderation and combining it with hydrating ingredients can help balance the skin's oil production without causing excessive dryness.

3. **Normal Skin**: Lemon peel powder can be used by individuals with normal skin types, but it's essential to monitor the skin's response. It can help maintain a healthy complexion by providing gentle exfoliation, brightening the skin tone, and controlling oiliness in the T-zone area.

4. **Sensitive Skin**: Individuals with sensitive skin should use lemon peel powder with caution, as it may cause irritation or redness, especially when used in high concentrations or on broken or inflamed skin. Performing a patch test before using lemon peel powder extensively is recommended to assess tolerance.

5. **Dry Skin**: Lemon peel powder may be too drying for individuals with dry or dehydrated skin, particularly when used alone or in high concentrations. However, it can still be incorporated into skincare routines in small amounts and combined with moisturizing ingredients to prevent excessive dryness.

6. **Acne-Prone Skin**: Lemon peel powder's antibacterial and exfoliating properties make it suitable for acne-prone skin. It helps unclog pores, reduce acne breakouts, and fade acne scars. However, individuals with acne-prone skin should be cautious and avoid overusing lemon peel powder, as it may exacerbate irritation or inflammation.

Overall, while lemon peel powder offers various benefits for the skin, its suitability depends on individual skin type and tolerance. It's essential to use lemon peel powder in moderation, perform a patch test before use, and discontinue use if any adverse reactions occur. If you have specific skin concerns or conditions, consult with a dermatologist or skincare professional for personalized recommendations.

Benefits of lemon peel powder

Lemon peel powder, derived from dried lemon peels, is packed with nutrients and natural compounds that offer numerous benefits for skincare. Here are some of the key benefits of lemon peel powder:

1. **Exfoliation**: Lemon peel powder has a slightly coarse texture, making it an effective natural exfoliant. It helps remove dead skin cells, dirt, and impurities from the skin's surface, revealing smoother, brighter, and more radiant skin underneath.

2. **Brightening**: Lemon peel powder contains citric acid, vitamin C, and other antioxidants that help brighten the skin and even out the complexion. Regular use of lemon peel powder can help lighten dark spots, hyperpigmentation, and acne scars, resulting in a more luminous and youthful appearance.

3. **Cleansing**: Lemon peel powder acts as a natural cleanser, effectively removing excess oil, dirt, and makeup residues from the skin. It helps unclog pores, prevent acne breakouts, and promote clearer and healthier-looking skin.

4. **Oil Control**: Lemon peel powder has astringent properties that help control excess oil production on the skin's surface. It helps mattify the complexion, reduce shine, and minimize the appearance of enlarged pores, making it beneficial for oily and acne-prone skin types.

5. **Antioxidant Protection**: Lemon peel powder is rich in antioxidants, including vitamin C, flavonoids, and polyphenols, which help protect the skin from oxidative stress and environmental damage caused by free radicals. Antioxidants help prevent premature aging signs such as fine lines, wrinkles, and sagging skin.

6. **Anti-inflammatory**: Lemon peel powder has anti-inflammatory properties that help soothe irritated or

inflamed skin. It can help reduce redness, itching, and inflammation associated with acne, eczema, sunburn, and other skin conditions.

7. **Skin Lightening**: Lemon peel powder contains natural bleaching agents that help lighten skin pigmentation and discoloration. It can be used to brighten dark spots, elbows, knees, and underarms, as well as to fade suntan and promote a more even skin tone.

8. **Refreshing**: Lemon peel powder has a refreshing and invigorating scent that uplifts the mood and rejuvenates the senses. It can be added to homemade skincare products like scrubs, masks, and bath salts for a spa-like experience.

9. **Hair Care**: Lemon peel powder can also benefit hair health by promoting scalp health, reducing dandruff, and adding shine to the hair. It can be used in homemade hair masks or rinses to nourish and strengthen the hair strands.

Overall, lemon peel powder is a versatile skincare ingredient that offers a wide range of benefits for the skin and hair. Whether used alone or in combination with other natural ingredients, lemon peel powder can help improve the overall health and appearance of the skin and hair.

Side effects of lemon peel powder

While lemon peel powder offers numerous benefits for skincare, it's essential to be aware of potential side effects and considerations, especially for individuals with sensitive skin. Here are some possible side effects of lemon peel powder:

1. **Skin Irritation**: Lemon peel powder contains citric acid and can be acidic, which may cause irritation, redness, or stinging sensation, particularly for those with sensitive or broken skin. Applying lemon peel powder

directly to the skin or using it in high concentrations can increase the risk of irritation. It's important to dilute lemon peel powder with water or other soothing ingredients and perform a patch test before applying it to a larger area of the skin.

2. **Photosensitivity**: Lemon peel contains compounds called psoralens, which can increase the skin's sensitivity to sunlight and UV radiation. Prolonged sun exposure after using products containing lemon peel powder may lead to sunburn, hyperpigmentation, or other adverse reactions. It's advisable to use lemon peel powder-based products in the evening and apply sunscreen during the day to protect the skin.

3. **Dryness**: Lemon peel powder can have a drying effect on the skin, particularly when used in high concentrations or on dry or sensitive skin types. Excessive use of lemon peel powder or leaving it on the skin for too long may lead to dryness, tightness, or flakiness. It's essential to moisturize the skin adequately after using products containing lemon peel powder to maintain skin hydration.

4. **Allergic Reactions**: Some individuals may be allergic to components in lemon peel powder, such as citric acid or limonene. Allergic reactions can manifest as itching, swelling, redness, hives, or rash. If you have known allergies to citrus fruits or sensitive skin, it's advisable to perform a patch test before using products containing lemon peel powder and discontinue use if any adverse reactions occur.

5. **Eye Irritation**: Avoid getting lemon peel powder or products containing it into the eyes, as it can cause irritation, stinging, or discomfort. If accidental contact occurs, rinse thoroughly with water and seek medical attention if irritation persists.

6. **Exacerbation of Certain Skin Conditions**: Individuals with certain skin conditions such as eczema, rosacea, or open wounds should use lemon peel powder with caution, as it may exacerbate existing inflammation or irritation. Consulting with a dermatologist before incorporating lemon peel powder into skincare routines is advisable, especially for those with sensitive or problematic skin.

Overall, while lemon peel powder can offer benefits for skincare, it's essential to use it cautiously and be mindful of potential side effects, especially for individuals with sensitive skin or allergies. If you experience any adverse reactions after using products containing lemon peel powder, discontinue use and consult with a dermatologist or healthcare professional for further guidance.

Different types of face pack can be prepared with lemon peel powder.

Certainly! Lemon peel powder can be used to create various DIY face packs that cater to different skin types and concerns. Here are some types of face packs you can prepare using lemon peel powder:

1. **Brightening Face Pack**:
    - Ingredients:
        - 2 tablespoons lemon peel powder
        - 1 tablespoon yogurt
        - 1 teaspoon honey
    - Instructions: Mix all the ingredients to form a paste. Apply the pack to cleansed skin and leave it on for 15-20 minutes. Rinse off with lukewarm water. This pack helps brighten the complexion and even out skin tone.

2. **Exfoliating Face Pack**:
    - Ingredients:

- 2 tablespoons lemon peel powder
- 1 tablespoon oatmeal
- 1 tablespoon honey

- Instructions: Mix all the ingredients to form a paste. Gently massage onto damp skin in circular motions for 1-2 minutes, then leave it on for an additional 10-15 minutes. Rinse off with water. This pack helps remove dead skin cells and reveal smoother skin.

3. **Acne-Fighting Face Pack**:
   - Ingredients:
     - 2 tablespoons lemon peel powder
     - 1 tablespoon neem powder
     - 1 tablespoon rose water.

   - Instructions: Mix all the ingredients to form a paste. Apply the pack to the face, focusing on acne-prone areas. Leave it on for 15-20 minutes, then rinse off with water. This pack helps control excess oil, reduce acne, and prevent breakouts.

4. **Hydrating Face Pack**:
   - Ingredients:
     - 2 tablespoons lemon peel powder
     - 1 tablespoon mashed avocado
     - 1 teaspoon almond oil

   - Instructions: Mix all the ingredients to form a creamy paste. Apply the pack to the face and leave it on for 20-30 minutes. Rinse off with lukewarm water. This pack helps moisturize and nourish dry skin.

5. **Toning Face Pack**:
   - Ingredients:

- 2 tablespoons lemon peel powder

- 1 tablespoon cucumber juice

- 1 teaspoon rose water.

- Instructions: Mix all the ingredients to form a paste. Apply it to the face and leave it on for 15-20 minutes. Rinse off with water. This pack helps tone and tighten the skin, reducing the appearance of pores.

6. **Soothing Face Pack**:
   - Ingredients:
     - 2 tablespoons lemon peel powder

     - 1 tablespoon aloe vera gel

     - 1 teaspoon coconut oil

   - Instructions: Mix all the ingredients to form a paste. Apply the pack to the face and leave it on for 15-20 minutes. Rinse off with water. This pack helps soothe irritated or inflamed skin.

These are just a few examples of face packs you can create using lemon peel powder. Feel free to customize the recipes based on your skin type and specific concerns. Always perform a patch test before using any new skincare product containing lemon peel powder to ensure compatibility and minimize the risk of irritation or allergic reactions.

Anar Peel Powder

Introduction to Anar peel powder

Anar peel powder, also known as pomegranate peel powder, is made from dried pomegranate peels and is renowned for its skincare benefits. Here are some of the key benefits of Anar peel powder:

1. **Exfoliation**: Anar peel powder has a slightly gritty texture, making it an excellent natural exfoliant. It helps remove dead skin cells, dirt, and impurities from the

skin's surface, leaving it smooth and refreshed.

2. **Anti-inflammatory**: Anar peel powder contains antioxidants and anti-inflammatory properties that help soothe irritated or inflamed skin. It can reduce redness, itching, and inflammation associated with acne, eczema, or sunburn.

3. **Brightening**: Anar peel powder is rich in vitamin C, which helps brighten the complexion and even out skin tone. Regular use of Anar peel powder can help fade dark spots, hyperpigmentation, and acne scars, resulting in a more radiant complexion.

4. **Cleansing**: Anar peel powder acts as a natural cleanser, effectively removing excess oil, dirt, and impurities from the skin. It helps unclog pores, prevent acne breakouts, and promote clearer and healthier-looking skin.

5. **Antioxidant Protection**: Anar peel powder is loaded with antioxidants, including polyphenols and flavonoids, which help protect the skin from oxidative stress and free radical damage. Antioxidants help prevent premature aging signs such as fine lines, wrinkles, and sagging skin.

6. **Oil Control**: Anar peel powder has astringent properties that help control excess oil production on the skin's surface. It helps mattify the complexion, reduce shine, and minimize the appearance of enlarged pores, making it beneficial for oily and acne-prone skin types.

7. **Skin Healing**: Anar peel powder contains compounds that promote skin regeneration and repair. It can accelerate the healing process of wounds, cuts, or minor skin irritations, leaving the skin looking healthy and rejuvenated.

8. **Anti-aging**: Regular use of Anar peel powder can

help stimulate collagen production and improve skin elasticity, reducing the appearance of fine lines and wrinkles. It helps maintain a youthful and firm complexion over time.

9. **Moisturizing**: Anar peel powder can help hydrate and moisturize the skin, leaving it soft, supple, and nourished. It can be combined with hydrating ingredients like honey, yogurt, or rose water to create moisturizing face masks or scrubs.

Overall, Anar peel powder is a versatile skincare ingredient that offers a wide range of benefits for the skin. Whether used alone or in combination with other natural ingredients, Anar peel powder can help improve the overall health and appearance of the skin, leaving it radiant, smooth, and youthful looking.

Anar peel powder suitable for which skin type

Pomegranate peel powder, also known as Anar peel powder, can offer benefits for various skin types, but its suitability may vary depending on individual skin concerns and sensitivities. Here's a breakdown of its suitability for different skin types:

1. **Normal Skin**: Pomegranate peel powder is generally suitable for normal skin types. It provides gentle exfoliation, helps brighten the complexion, and promotes overall skin health. Normal skin types can benefit from the antioxidant-rich properties of pomegranate peel powder to maintain a youthful and radiant complexion.

2. **Oily Skin**: Pomegranate peel powder is beneficial for oily skin types due to its astringent properties. It helps control excess oil production, reduce shine, and minimize the appearance of enlarged pores. The exfoliating action of pomegranate peel powder also helps unclog pores and prevent acne breakouts, making it suitable for oily and acne-prone skin.

3. **Combination Skin**: Individuals with combination skin can also benefit from using pomegranate peel powder, but they should be mindful of potential dryness in drier areas of the face. Pomegranate peel powder helps balance oil production, exfoliate the skin, and promote a more even complexion. Using it in combination with hydrating ingredients can help maintain skin balance.

4. **Dry Skin**: While pomegranate peel powder offers exfoliating and brightening benefits, it may be too drying for individuals with dry or sensitive skin. Pomegranate peel powder can exacerbate dryness or irritation, particularly when used in high concentrations or on sensitive areas. Dry skin types may prefer to use pomegranate peel powder in moderation and combine it with moisturizing ingredients to prevent excessive dryness.

5. **Sensitive Skin**: Individuals with sensitive skin should use pomegranate peel powder with caution, as it may cause irritation or redness, especially when used in high concentrations or on broken or inflamed skin. Performing a patch test before using pomegranate peel powder extensively is recommended to assess tolerance. Sensitive skin types may benefit from using pomegranate peel powder in diluted forms or incorporating it into gentle skincare formulations.

Overall, while pomegranate peel powder offers various skincare benefits, its suitability depends on individual skin type, concerns, and tolerance. It's essential to monitor the skin's response and adjust usage accordingly. If you have specific skin concerns or conditions, consulting with a dermatologist or skincare professional before incorporating pomegranate peel powder into your skincare routine is advisable for personalized recommendations.

Benefits of Anar peel powder

Pomegranate peel powder, also known as Anar peel powder, offers a variety of benefits for skin and hair care due to its rich nutrient content and natural properties. Here are some of the key benefits of Anar peel powder:

1. **Exfoliation**: Anar peel powder has a slightly coarse texture, making it an effective natural exfoliant. It helps remove dead skin cells, dirt, and impurities from the skin's surface, revealing smoother and brighter skin underneath.

2. **Antioxidant Protection**: Pomegranate peel powder is rich in antioxidants, including flavonoids, polyphenols, and vitamin C. These antioxidants help protect the skin from oxidative stress and free radical damage, which can lead to premature aging signs such as fine lines, wrinkles, and sagging skin.

3. **Brightening**: The vitamin C content in pomegranate peel powder helps brighten the complexion and even out skin tone. Regular use of Anar peel powder can help fade dark spots, hyperpigmentation, and acne scars, resulting in a more radiant and youthful appearance.

4. **Anti-inflammatory**: Pomegranate peel powder contains anti-inflammatory properties that help soothe irritated or inflamed skin. It can reduce redness, itching, and inflammation associated with acne, eczema, or sunburn.

5. **Oil Control**: Anar peel powder has astringent properties that help control excess oil production on the skin's surface. It helps mattify the complexion, reduce shine, and minimize the appearance of enlarged pores, making it beneficial for oily and acne-prone skin types.

6. **Anti-aging**: Regular use of pomegranate peel powder can help stimulate collagen production and improve skin elasticity, reducing the appearance of fine lines

and wrinkles. It helps maintain a youthful and firm complexion over time.

7. **Cleansing**: Pomegranate peel powder acts as a natural cleanser, effectively removing excess oil, dirt, and impurities from the skin. It helps unclog pores, prevent acne breakouts, and promote clearer and healthier-looking skin.

8. **Hydrating**: Anar peel powder can help hydrate and moisturize the skin, leaving it soft, supple, and nourished. It can be combined with hydrating ingredients like honey, yogurt, or rose water to create moisturizing face masks or scrubs.

9. **Hair Care**: Pomegranate peel powder can also benefit hair health by promoting scalp health, reducing dandruff, and adding shine to the hair. It can be used in homemade hair masks or rinses to nourish and strengthen the hair strands.

Overall, Anar peel powder is a versatile skincare ingredient that offers a wide range of benefits for the skin and hair. Whether used alone or in combination with other natural ingredients, pomegranate peel powder can help improve the overall health and appearance of the skin and hair, leaving them looking radiant, smooth, and youthful.

Side effects of Anar peel powder

While Anar peel powder offers numerous benefits for skin and hair care, it's essential to be aware of potential side effects and considerations, especially for individuals with sensitive skin or specific allergies. Here are some possible side effects of Anar peel powder:

1. **Skin Irritation**: Anar peel powder may cause skin irritation, redness, or itching, particularly for individuals with sensitive skin or those prone to

allergies. Direct application of undiluted Anar peel powder or using it in high concentrations can increase the risk of irritation. It's advisable to perform a patch test before applying Anar peel powder extensively to assess skin sensitivity.

2. **Photosensitivity**: Pomegranate peel contains compounds that may increase the skin's sensitivity to sunlight and UV radiation. Prolonged sun exposure after using products containing Anar peel powder may lead to sunburn, hyperpigmentation, or other adverse reactions. It's essential to use sunscreen and avoid excessive sun exposure after using Anar peel powder-based products.

3. **Dryness**: Anar peel powder has astringent properties that can potentially cause dryness, particularly for individuals with dry or sensitive skin. Using Anar peel powder in high concentrations or leaving it on the skin for too long may lead to dryness, tightness, or flakiness. It's important to moisturize the skin adequately after using products containing Anar peel powder to maintain skin hydration.

4. **Allergic Reactions**: Some individuals may be allergic to components in Anar peel powder, such as polyphenols or other bioactive compounds. Allergic reactions can manifest as itching, swelling, redness, hives, or rash. If you have known allergies to pomegranate or sensitive skin, it's advisable to perform a patch test before using Anar peel powder extensively and discontinue use if any adverse reactions occur.

5. **Eye Irritation**: Avoid getting Anar peel powder or products containing it into the eyes, as it can cause irritation, stinging, or discomfort. If accidental contact occurs, rinse thoroughly with water and seek medical attention if irritation persists.

6. **Exacerbation of Certain Skin Conditions**: Individuals with certain skin conditions such as eczema, rosacea, or open wounds should use Anar peel powder with caution, as it may exacerbate existing inflammation or irritation. Consulting with a dermatologist before incorporating Anar peel powder into skincare routines is advisable, especially for those with sensitive or problematic skin.

Overall, while Anar peel powder offers various skincare benefits, its suitability depends on individual skin type, concerns, and tolerance. It's essential to monitor the skin's response and discontinue use if any adverse reactions occur. If you have specific skin concerns or conditions, consulting with a dermatologist or skincare professional before using Anar peel powder is recommended for personalized recommendations.

Different types of face pack can be prepared with Anar peel powder.

Certainly! Pomegranate peel powder, also known as Anar peel powder, can be used to create various DIY face packs that cater to different skin types and concerns. Here are some types of face packs you can prepare using Anar peel powder:

1. **Brightening Face Pack**:
   - Ingredients:
     - 2 tablespoons Anar peel powder
     - 1 tablespoon yogurt
     - 1 teaspoon honey
   - Instructions: Mix all the ingredients to form a paste. Apply the pack to cleansed skin and leave it on for 15-20 minutes. Rinse off with lukewarm water. This pack helps brighten the complexion and even out skin tone.

2. **Exfoliating Face Pack**:

- Ingredients:
    - 2 tablespoons Anar peel powder
    - 1 tablespoon oatmeal
    - 1 tablespoon rose water.
- Instructions: Mix all the ingredients to form a paste. Gently massage onto damp skin in circular motions for 1-2 minutes, then leave it on for an additional 10-15 minutes. Rinse off with water. This pack helps remove dead skin cells and reveal smoother skin.

3. **Hydrating Face Pack**:
    - Ingredients:
        - 2 tablespoons Anar peel powder
        - 1 tablespoon mashed avocado
        - 1 teaspoon almond oil
    - Instructions: Mix all the ingredients to form a creamy paste. Apply the pack to the face and leave it on for 20-30 minutes. Rinse off with lukewarm water. This pack helps moisturize and nourish dry skin.

4. **Anti-aging Face Pack**:
    - Ingredients:
        - 2 tablespoons Anar peel powder
        - 1 tablespoon rose water.
        - 1 teaspoon honey
    - Instructions: Mix all the ingredients to form a paste. Apply the pack to the face and leave it on for 15-20 minutes. Rinse off with water. This pack helps stimulate collagen production, improve skin elasticity, and reduce the appearance of fine lines and wrinkles.

5. **Acne-Fighting Face Pack**:

- Ingredients:
    - 2 tablespoons Anar peel powder
    - 1 tablespoon neem powder
    - 1 tablespoon rose water.
- Instructions: Mix all the ingredients to form a paste. Apply the pack to the face, focusing on acne-prone areas. Leave it on for 15-20 minutes, then rinse off with water. This pack helps control excess oil, reduce acne, and prevent breakouts.

6. **Soothing Face Pack**:
    - Ingredients:
        - 2 tablespoons anar peel powder
        - 1 tablespoon aloe vera gel
        - 1 teaspoon coconut oil
    - Instructions: Mix all the ingredients to form a paste. Apply the pack to the face and leave it on for 15-20 minutes. Rinse off with water. This pack helps soothe irritated or inflamed skin.

These are just a few examples of face packs you can create using Anar peel powder. Feel free to customize the recipes based on your skin type and specific concerns. Always perform a patch test before using any new skincare product containing Anar peel powder to ensure compatibility and minimize the risk of irritation or allergic reactions.

Masoor Dal Powder

Introduction to masoor dal powder

Masoor dal powder, derived from dried and powdered red lentils, is a versatile ingredient used in skincare for its various benefits. Here are some of the potential benefits of masoor dal powder for the skin:

1. **Exfoliation**: Masoor dal powder has a slightly gritty texture, making it an effective natural exfoliant. It helps remove dead skin cells, dirt, and impurities from the

skin's surface, leaving it smooth and refreshed.

2. **Brightening**: The presence of vitamins and minerals in masoor dal powder, such as vitamin B, iron, and potassium, can help brighten the complexion and even out skin tone. Regular use of masoor dal powder can impart a radiant glow to the skin.

3. **Oil Control**: Masoor dal powder possesses absorbent properties that help absorb excess oil from the skin's surface. It can be beneficial for individuals with oily or combination skin types by helping to mattify the complexion and reduce shine.

4. **Acne Treatment**: Masoor dal powder has anti-inflammatory and antimicrobial properties that can help in the treatment of acne. It helps soothe inflammation, reduce redness, and prevent further breakouts when used regularly.

5. **Skin Tightening**: The astringent properties of masoor dal powder can help tighten and firm the skin, reducing the appearance of enlarged pores and improving skin texture.

6. **Anti-aging**: Masoor dal powder contains antioxidants that help fight free radicals and prevent oxidative stress, which can contribute to premature aging signs such as fine lines and wrinkles. Regular use may help promote youthful-looking skin.

7. **Scar Reduction**: Masoor dal powder can help fade scars and blemishes over time with its exfoliating and skin-brightening properties. It aids in the removal of dead skin cells and promotes cell turnover, leading to the gradual lightening of scars.

8. **Soothing**: Masoor dal powder has a cooling effect on the skin, making it suitable for soothing sunburns, irritation, or inflammation. It helps calm the skin and

provides relief from discomfort.

9. **Nourishment**: Masoor dal powder contains nutrients that nourish the skin, keeping it healthy and supple. It can help maintain the skin's moisture balance and prevent dryness.

10. **Detoxification**: Masoor dal powder can assist in detoxifying the skin by removing toxins, impurities, and excess sebum, resulting in clearer and healthier-looking skin.

Overall, masoor dal powder offers numerous benefits for skincare and can be incorporated into various DIY face packs, scrubs, and masks to promote healthier, glowing skin.

Masoor dal powder suitable for which skin type

Masoor dal powder is generally suitable for most skin types, but its effectiveness and recommended usage may vary depending on individual skin concerns and conditions. Here's a breakdown of its suitability for different skin types:

1. **Normal Skin**: Masoor dal powder can be beneficial for normal skin types as it offers gentle exfoliation, brightening, and oil-absorbing properties. It helps maintain the skin's texture, improves complexion, and removes impurities without causing excessive dryness or irritation.

2. **Oily Skin**: Masoor dal powder is particularly suitable for oily and combination skin types. Its absorbent properties help control excess oil production, reduce shine, and prevent clogged pores. Regular use can help mattify the complexion and minimize the appearance of enlarged pores, making it an effective ingredient in managing oily skin.

3. **Combination Skin**: Individuals with combination skin can also benefit from masoor dal powder, but they

may need to adjust its usage based on specific areas of concern. It can be used on oily areas to control sebum production and as a spot treatment on acne-prone areas. However, caution should be taken to prevent over-drying of dry or sensitive areas.

4. **Dry Skin**: Masoor dal powder may not be as suitable for individuals with dry or sensitive skin types, as it can potentially exacerbate dryness or irritation. However, when used in moderation and combined with moisturizing ingredients such as honey, yogurt, or milk, it can provide gentle exfoliation and nourishment to dry skin without stripping away moisture.

5. **Sensitive Skin**: Individuals with sensitive skin should use masoor dal powder with caution, as its coarse texture may cause irritation or redness, especially when used aggressively. Performing a patch test before applying masoor dal powder to larger areas of the skin is recommended to assess sensitivity. Additionally, using finely ground masoor dal powder or incorporating it into mild formulations may help minimize the risk of irritation.

6. **Acne-Prone Skin**: Masoor dal powder can be beneficial for acne-prone skin due to its exfoliating and oil-absorbing properties. It helps unclog pores, remove dead skin cells, and reduce the occurrence of breakouts. However, individuals with acne-prone skin should avoid excessive scrubbing and ensure proper hydration after using masoor dal powder to prevent over-drying.

Overall, while masoor dal powder offers various skincare benefits, its suitability depends on individual skin type, concerns, and tolerance. It's essential to monitor the skin's response and adjust usage accordingly. If you have specific skin concerns or conditions, consulting with a dermatologist or skincare professional before incorporating masoor dal powder into your skincare routine is advisable for personalized recommendations.

Benefits of masoor dal powder

Masoor dal powder, derived from dried and powdered red lentils, is a versatile ingredient that offers numerous benefits for skincare. Here are some of the key benefits of masoor dal powder:

1. **Exfoliation**: Masoor dal powder has a slightly coarse texture, making it an effective natural exfoliant. It helps remove dead skin cells, dirt, and impurities from the skin's surface, revealing smoother and brighter skin underneath.

2. **Oil Control**: Masoor dal powder possesses absorbent properties that help control excess oil production on the skin's surface. It can be beneficial for individuals with oily or combination skin types by helping to mattify the complexion and reduce shine.

3. **Brightening**: The presence of vitamins and minerals in masoor dal powder, such as vitamin B, iron, and potassium, can help brighten the complexion and even out skin tone. Regular use of masoor dal powder can impart a radiant glow to the skin.

4. **Acne Treatment**: Masoor dal powder has anti-inflammatory and antimicrobial properties that can help in the treatment of acne. It helps soothe inflammation, reduce redness, and prevent further breakouts when used regularly.

5. **Skin Tightening**: The astringent properties of masoor dal powder can help tighten and firm the skin, reducing the appearance of enlarged pores and improving skin texture.

6. **Anti-aging**: Masoor dal powder contains antioxidants

that help fight free radicals and prevent oxidative stress, which can contribute to premature aging signs such as fine lines and wrinkles. Regular use may help promote youthful-looking skin.

7. **Scar Reduction**: Masoor dal powder can help fade scars and blemishes over time with its exfoliating and skin-brightening properties. It aids in the removal of dead skin cells and promotes cell turnover, leading to the gradual lightening of scars.

8. **Soothing**: Masoor dal powder has a cooling effect on the skin, making it suitable for soothing sunburns, irritation, or inflammation. It helps calm the skin and provides relief from discomfort.

9. **Nourishment**: Masoor dal powder contains nutrients that nourish the skin, keeping it healthy and supple. It can help maintain the skin's moisture balance and prevent dryness.

10. **Detoxification**: Masoor dal powder can assist in detoxifying the skin by removing toxins, impurities, and excess sebum, resulting in clearer and healthier-looking skin.

Overall, masoor dal powder offers a range of benefits for skincare and can be incorporated into various DIY face packs, scrubs, and masks to promote healthier, glowing skin.

Side effects of masoor dal powder

While masoor dal powder offers numerous benefits for skincare, it's essential to be aware of potential side effects and considerations, especially for individuals with sensitive skin or specific allergies. Here are some possible side effects of masoor dal powder:

1. **Skin Irritation**: Masoor dal powder has a coarse texture, which can potentially cause irritation, redness, or itching, particularly for individuals with sensitive skin. Direct application of undiluted masoor dal powder or using it in high concentrations can increase the risk of irritation. It's advisable to perform a patch test before applying masoor dal powder extensively to assess skin sensitivity.

2. **Allergic Reactions**: Some individuals may be allergic to components in masoor dal powder, such as proteins or other compounds present in lentils. Allergic reactions can manifest as itching, swelling, redness, hives, or rash. If you have known allergies to legumes or sensitive skin, it's advisable to perform a patch test before using masoor dal powder extensively and discontinue use if any adverse reactions occur.

3. **Dryness**: Masoor dal powder has absorbent properties that can potentially cause dryness, particularly for individuals with dry or sensitive skin types. Using masoor dal powder in high concentrations or leaving it on the skin for too long may lead to dryness, tightness, or flakiness. It's important to moisturize the skin adequately after using masoor dal powder to maintain skin hydration.

4. **Exacerbation of Certain Skin Conditions**: Individuals with certain skin conditions such as eczema, rosacea, or open wounds should use masoor dal powder with caution, as it may exacerbate existing inflammation or irritation. Consulting with a dermatologist before incorporating masoor dal powder into skincare routines is advisable, especially for those with sensitive or problematic skin.

5. **Eye Irritation**: Avoid getting masoor dal powder or products containing it into the eyes, as it can cause

irritation, stinging, or discomfort. If accidental contact occurs, rinse thoroughly with water and seek medical attention if irritation persists.

6. **Digestive Issues (if ingested)**: While the focus here is on topical use, it's worth noting that masoor dal powder is primarily used in cooking. Ingestion of large amounts of masoor dal powder may cause digestive discomfort or allergic reactions in some individuals, particularly those with sensitivities to legumes.

Overall, while masoor dal powder offers various skincare benefits, its suitability depends on individual skin type, concerns, and tolerance. It's essential to monitor the skin's response and discontinue use if any adverse reactions occur. If you have specific skin concerns or conditions, consulting with a dermatologist or skincare professional before using masoor dal powder is recommended for personalized recommendations.

Different types of face pack can be prepared with masoor dal powder.

Masoor dal powder is a versatile ingredient that can be used to create various DIY face packs tailored to different skin types and concerns. Here are some types of face packs you can prepare using masoor dal powder:

1. **Brightening Face Pack**:
   - Ingredients:
     - 2 tablespoons masoor dal powder
     - 1 tablespoon yogurt
     - 1 teaspoon honey
   - Instructions: Mix all the ingredients to form a paste. Apply the pack to cleansed skin and leave it on for 15-20 minutes. Rinse off with lukewarm water. This pack helps brighten the complexion and even out skin tone.

2. **Exfoliating Face Pack**:
   - Ingredients:
     - 2 tablespoons masoor dal powder
     - 1 tablespoon oatmeal
     - 1 tablespoon rose water.
   - Instructions: Mix all the ingredients to form a paste. Gently massage onto damp skin in circular motions for 1-2 minutes, then leave it on for an additional 10-15 minutes. Rinse off with water. This pack helps remove dead skin cells and reveal smoother skin.

3. **Hydrating Face Pack**:
   - Ingredients:
     - 2 tablespoons masoor dal powder
     - 1 tablespoon mashed avocado
     - 1 teaspoon almond oil
   - Instructions: Mix all the ingredients to form a creamy paste. Apply the pack to the face and leave it on for 20-30 minutes. Rinse off with lukewarm water. This pack helps moisturize and nourish dry skin.

4. **Acne-Fighting Face Pack**:
   - Ingredients:
     - 2 tablespoons masoor dal powder
     - 1 tablespoon neem powder
     - 1 tablespoon rose water.
   - Instructions: Mix all the ingredients to form a paste. Apply the pack to the face, focusing on acne-prone areas. Leave it on for 15-20 minutes, then rinse off with water. This pack helps control excess oil, reduce acne, and prevent breakouts.

5. **Soothing Face Pack**:
    - Ingredients:
        - 2 tablespoons masoor dal powder
        - 1 tablespoon aloe vera gel
        - 1 teaspoon coconut oil
    - Instructions: Mix all the ingredients to form a paste. Apply the pack to the face and leave it on for 15-20 minutes. Rinse off with water. This pack helps soothe irritated or inflamed skin.

6. **Skin Tightening Face Pack**:
    - Ingredients:
        - 2 tablespoons masoor dal powder
        - 1 egg white
        - 1 teaspoon lemon juice
    - Instructions: Mix all the ingredients to form a paste. Apply the pack to the face and leave it on for 15-20 minutes. Rinse off with water. This pack helps tighten and firm the skin, reducing the appearance of enlarged pores.

These are just a few examples of face packs you can create using masoor dal powder. Feel free to customize the recipes based on your skin type and specific concerns. Always perform a patch test before using any new skincare product containing masoor dal powder to ensure compatibility and minimize the risk of irritation or allergic reactions.

Potato Powder

Introduction to potato powder

Potato powder, made from dried and ground potatoes, is a versatile ingredient that offers various benefits for skincare. Here are some of the key benefits of potato powder:

1. **Brightening**: Potato powder contains enzymes, vitamins (such as vitamin C), and minerals that help brighten the skin and even out skin tone. Regular use can diminish the appearance of dark spots, hyperpigmentation, and dullness, resulting in a more radiant complexion.

2. **Soothing**: Potato powder has anti-inflammatory properties that help soothe irritated or inflamed skin. It can provide relief from conditions such as sunburn, rashes, and insect bites, leaving the skin feeling calmer and more comfortable.

3. **Hydrating**: Potato powder has moisturizing properties that help hydrate the skin, making it softer, smoother, and more supple. It can be beneficial for individuals with dry or dehydrated skin, providing an extra boost of hydration.

4. **Oil Control**: Potato powder can help absorb excess oil from the skin's surface, making it beneficial for individuals with oily or combination skin types. It helps mattify the complexion, reduce shine, and minimize the appearance of enlarged pores.

5. **Anti-aging**: Potato powder contains antioxidants, such

as vitamin C, that help fight free radicals and prevent oxidative stress, which can contribute to premature aging signs such as fine lines and wrinkles. Regular use may help promote youthful-looking skin.

6. **Exfoliation**: Potato powder has a slightly gritty texture, making it an effective natural exfoliant. It helps remove dead skin cells, dirt, and impurities from the skin's surface, revealing smoother and brighter skin underneath.

7. **Acne Treatment**: Potato powder has antibacterial properties that can help in the treatment of acne. It helps cleanse the skin, unclog pores, and reduce the occurrence of breakouts. It can also help soothe acne-related inflammation and redness.

8. **Skin Lightening**: Potato powder contains enzymes that may help lighten and fade dark spots, acne scars, and blemishes over time. It promotes cell turnover and renewal, resulting in a more even complexion.

9. **Cooling Effect**: Potato powder has a cooling effect on the skin, making it suitable for soothing sunburns, irritation, or heat-related discomfort. It helps refresh and revitalize the skin, providing instant relief.

Overall, potato powder offers a range of benefits for skincare and can be incorporated into various DIY face masks, scrubs, and treatments to promote healthier, glowing skin.

Potato powder suitable for which skin type

Potato powder is generally suitable for various skin types, but its effectiveness and recommended usage may vary depending on individual skin concerns and conditions. Here's a breakdown of its suitability for different skin types:

1. **Normal Skin**: Potato powder can be beneficial for normal skin types as it offers brightening, soothing, and

hydrating properties. It helps even out skin tone, reduce inflammation, and provide lightweight hydration without clogging pores.

2. **Oily Skin**: Potato powder is particularly suitable for oily and combination skin types. Its oil-absorbing properties help control excess sebum production, reduce shine, and minimize the appearance of enlarged pores. Regular use can help mattify the complexion and prevent breakouts.

3. **Combination Skin**: Individuals with combination skin can also benefit from potato powder, but they may need to adjust its usage based on specific areas of concern. It can be used on oily areas to control oiliness and as a spot treatment on dry or sensitive areas to provide hydration without exacerbating oiliness.

4. **Dry Skin**: While potato powder may not provide intense hydration for dry skin on its own, it can be incorporated into moisturizing face masks or treatments to add a soothing and brightening effect. When combined with hydrating ingredients like honey, yogurt, or avocado, potato powder can help nourish and soften dry skin.

5. **Sensitive Skin**: Potato powder is generally well-tolerated by sensitive skin types due to its natural and gentle properties. It helps soothe irritation, reduce redness, and provide relief from inflammation without causing further sensitivity. However, individuals with specific allergies or sensitivities should perform a patch test before using potato powder extensively.

6. **Acne-Prone Skin**: Potato powder can be beneficial for acne-prone skin due to its anti-inflammatory and antibacterial properties. It helps cleanse the skin, unclog pores, and reduce acne-related inflammation and redness. Regular use may help prevent breakouts and promote clearer skin.

Overall, while potato powder offers various skincare benefits, its suitability depends on individual skin type, concerns, and tolerance. It's essential to monitor the skin's response and adjust usage accordingly. If you have specific skin concerns or conditions, consulting with a dermatologist or skincare professional before incorporating potato powder into your skincare routine is advisable for personalized recommendations.

Benefits of potato powder

Potato powder, derived from dried and ground potatoes, offers several benefits for skincare due to its nutrient-rich composition and natural properties. Here are some of the key benefits of potato powder:

1. **Brightening**: Potato powder contains enzymes, vitamins (such as vitamin C), and minerals that help brighten the skin and even out skin tone. Regular use can diminish the appearance of dark spots, hyperpigmentation, and dullness, resulting in a more radiant complexion.

2. **Soothing**: Potato powder has anti-inflammatory properties that help soothe irritated or inflamed skin. It can provide relief from conditions such as sunburn, rashes, and insect bites, leaving the skin feeling calmer and more comfortable.

3. **Hydrating**: Potato powder has moisturizing properties that help hydrate the skin, making it softer, smoother, and more supple. It can be beneficial for individuals with dry or dehydrated skin, providing an extra boost of hydration.

4. **Oil Control**: Potato powder can help absorb excess oil from the skin's surface, making it beneficial for individuals with oily or combination skin types. It helps

mattify the complexion, reduce shine, and minimize the appearance of enlarged pores.

5. **Anti-aging**: Potato powder contains antioxidants, such as vitamin C, that help fight free radicals and prevent oxidative stress, which can contribute to premature aging signs such as fine lines and wrinkles. Regular use may help promote youthful-looking skin.

6. **Exfoliation**: Potato powder has a slightly gritty texture, making it an effective natural exfoliant. It helps remove dead skin cells, dirt, and impurities from the skin's surface, revealing smoother and brighter skin underneath.

7. **Acne Treatment**: Potato powder has antibacterial properties that can help in the treatment of acne. It helps cleanse the skin, unclog pores, and reduce the occurrence of breakouts. It can also help soothe acne-related inflammation and redness.

8. **Skin Lightening**: Potato powder contains enzymes that may help lighten and fade dark spots, acne scars, and blemishes over time. It promotes cell turnover and renewal, resulting in a more even complexion.

9. **Cooling Effect**: Potato powder has a cooling effect on the skin, making it suitable for soothing sunburns, irritation, or heat-related discomfort. It helps refresh and revitalize the skin, providing instant relief.

Overall, potato powder offers a range of benefits for skincare and can be incorporated into various DIY face masks, scrubs, and treatments to promote healthier, glowing skin.

Side effects of potato powder

While potato powder offers numerous benefits for skincare, it's essential to be aware of potential side effects and considerations, especially for individuals with sensitive skin or specific allergies. Here are some possible side effects of potato powder:

1. **Skin Irritation**: Some individuals may experience skin irritation or allergic reactions when using potato powder topically. This can manifest as redness, itching, inflammation, or rash. It's essential to perform a patch test before applying potato powder extensively to assess skin sensitivity.

2. **Dryness**: Potato powder can have a drying effect on the skin, particularly when used in high concentrations or for an extended period. It may strip away natural oils, leading to dryness, tightness, or flakiness. Individuals with dry or sensitive skin should use potato powder with caution and ensure proper hydration after use.

3. **Exacerbation of Existing Skin Conditions**: Individuals with certain skin conditions such as eczema, psoriasis, or dermatitis may find that potato powder exacerbates their symptoms. It can potentially increase irritation, redness, or inflammation in sensitive or compromised skin. Consulting with a dermatologist before using potato powder is advisable for individuals with pre-existing skin conditions.

4. **Photosensitivity**: While not as common as with some other ingredients, potato powder may increase the skin's sensitivity to sunlight in some individuals. Prolonged sun exposure after using products containing potato powder may lead to sunburn or hyperpigmentation. It's essential to use sunscreen and avoid excessive sun exposure when using potato powder-based products.

5. **Allergic Reactions**: Individuals with allergies to potatoes or other related substances may experience allergic reactions when using potato powder. Symptoms

can include itching, swelling, hives, or difficulty breathing. It's crucial to discontinue use immediately and seek medical attention if allergic reactions occur.

6. **Eye Irritation**: Avoid getting potato powder or products containing it into the eyes, as it can cause irritation, stinging, or discomfort. If accidental contact occurs, rinse thoroughly with water and seek medical attention if irritation persists.

7. **Digestive Issues (if ingested)**: While the focus here is on topical use, it's worth noting that potato powder is primarily used in cooking. Ingestion of large amounts of potato powder may cause digestive discomfort or allergic reactions in some individuals, particularly those with sensitivities to potatoes.

Overall, while potato powder offers various skincare benefits, its suitability depends on individual skin type, concerns, and tolerance. It's essential to monitor the skin's response and discontinue use if any adverse reactions occur. If you have specific skin concerns or conditions, consulting with a dermatologist or skincare professional before using potato powder is recommended for personalized recommendations.

Different types of face pack can be prepared with potato powder.

Certainly! Potato powder can be used to create various DIY face packs tailored to different skin types and concerns. Here are some types of face packs you can prepare using potato powder:

1. **Brightening Face Pack**:
   - Ingredients:
     - 2 tablespoons potato powder
     - 1 tablespoon lemon juice
     - 1 tablespoon honey
   - Instructions: Mix all the ingredients to form a

smooth paste. Apply the pack to cleansed skin and leave it on for 15-20 minutes. Rinse off with lukewarm water. This pack helps brighten the complexion and reduce dark spots.

2. **Soothing Face Pack**:
   - Ingredients:
     - 2 tablespoons potato powder
     - 1 tablespoon yogurt
     - 1 teaspoon cucumber juice
   - Instructions: Mix all the ingredients to form a paste. Apply the pack to the face and leave it on for 15-20 minutes. Rinse off with water. This pack helps soothe irritated or inflamed skin and provides a cooling effect.

3. **Hydrating Face Pack**:
   - Ingredients:
     - 2 tablespoons potato powder
     - 1 tablespoon mashed avocado
     - 1 teaspoon almond oil
   - Instructions: Mix all the ingredients to form a creamy paste. Apply the pack to the face and leave it on for 20-30 minutes. Rinse off with lukewarm water. This pack helps moisturize and nourish dry skin.

4. **Exfoliating Face Pack**:
   - Ingredients:
     - 2 tablespoons potato powder
     - 1 tablespoon oatmeal
     - 1 tablespoon rose water.
   - Instructions: Mix all the ingredients to form a paste. Gently massage onto damp skin in circular motions for 1-2 minutes, then leave it

on for an additional 10-15 minutes. Rinse off with water. This pack helps remove dead skin cells and reveal smoother skin.

5. **Oil-Control Face Pack**:
    - Ingredients:
        - 2 tablespoons potato powder
        - 1 tablespoon fuller's earth (Multani Miti)
        - 1 tablespoon rose water.
    - Instructions: Mix all the ingredients to form a paste. Apply the pack to the face and leave it on until it dries. Rinse off with water. This pack helps absorb excess oil and tighten pores.

6. **Anti-Acne Face Pack**:
    - Ingredients:
        - 2 tablespoons potato powder
        - 1 tablespoon aloe vera gel
        - 1 teaspoon tea tree oil
    - Instructions: Mix all the ingredients to form a paste. Apply the pack to the face, focusing on acne-prone areas. Leave it on for 15-20 minutes, then rinse off with water. This pack helps reduce acne and soothe inflammation.

These are just a few examples of face packs you can create using potato powder. Feel free to customize the recipes based on your skin type and specific concerns. Always perform a patch test before using any new skincare product containing potato powder to ensure compatibility and minimize the risk of irritation or allergic reactions.

www.ingramcontent.com/pod-product-compliance
Lightning Source LLC
Chambersburg PA
CBHW072248260726
48659CB00004BA/1488